Praise for *Holding on in the Storm*

Clear, unsentimental writing, coupled with wise insights. *Holding on in the Storm* is not just about one husband's grief, but how he wrestled biblically in a culture whose approach to life issues seems so reasonable but is so often at odds with our faith. This makes it a perfect book for small group study—both an engaging, heartfelt story along with a clear-headed biblical understanding of suffering and death.
Mark Galli, former editor in chief at *Christianity Today*

It is impossible to read *Holding on in the Storm* without imagining yourself in the same situation as author Bob Cutillo and his wife Heather. What if I or my loved one receive a dismal diagnosis of stage 4 cancer? How would I respond? For people of faith, there is an even bigger question that looms above all others. Will I be faithful in the midst of this horrendous storm? We wonder if we have what it takes. Is our faith strong enough to endure the pain and grief?

The struggle to hang on to God's goodness in the tough realities of suffering is really nothing new. What is different is the author's willingness to be vulnerable in our modern cultural context. Cutillo's story inspires the reader because he risks sharing his innermost thoughts, beckoning the reader to come alongside him as he asks the difficult questions we are afraid to ask. It is a hard but holy journey, sprinkled with unexpected moments of grace. But if you are willing to open your heart to feel the ache, you too will likely feel the firm grasp of God in the storm.
Missy Buchanan, author of *Feeling Your Way through Grief*

Bob Cutillo's *Holding on in the Storm* caught me by surprise. I have read many books on loss, but none like his. On the surface he tells the story of his wife's experience of cancer, which resulted in her death in 2023. He tells that story not only through his own voice but also through hers, quoting extensively from her posts on the CaringBridge website. But there is more than surface to this book. The story serves as an example of what marriage should and can be, "in sickness and in health." It also demonstrates Cutillo's extraordinary capacity for reflection, which integrates personal insight, quotes from great authors like Dante, Donne, and Bonhoeffer, many Psalms, and the medical knowledge he acquired as a physician into a larger whole. It is obvious that Cutillo is anchored in the Christian faith as few people are. What emerges is a profound book about suffering and loss. It is starkly beautiful, like a winter landscape. It moved me, and it called forth life in me.

Jerry Sittser is a professor emeritus of theology and author of *A Grace Disguised* **and** *Water from a Deep Well*

I've learned that in the middle of our personal storms, we often feel like we're drowning. From my own experience, I know there are thousands of lifelines that can buoy us, that can help us tread water, if only for a while. The challenge is, during the storm, we're lost in an abyss of pain, confusion, and fog. What we need is someone to place the lifeline in our hands, around our waist, or under our arms. Grievers need a guide, a steady captain to guide the boat while we float toward safety.

Bob's story is that gentle guide. With tenderness and clarity, he invites us into his life with Heather—their Christ-centered marriage and their unwavering commitment to care for others. Bob's love for Heather, their mutual passion for service, and their deep trust in God's plan shines through every page. The personal stories shared—first by Heather and Bob together, then by Bob alone—are raw, emotional, and profoundly valuable to anyone navigating grief or supporting someone who is.

My own storm included the loss of my father and my oldest son in a hate crime. When Bob described feeling like a "dead man walking" after losing Heather, I felt the weight of those words in my bones. Reading *Holding on in the Storm* brought me comfort, even eleven years after my own loss. This empathetic, faith-filled message will do the same for you.

Mindy Corporon, author of *Healing a Shattered Soul, Leading through Grief,* **and the co-founder of SevenDays Inc. and Workplace Healing Inc.**

With *Holding on in the Storm*, Bob Cutillo invites the reader to join him as he reveals his story of suffering, but even more so reveals the deeper reality of the anguish that each of us will invariably encounter. The anguish of fear, pain, and suffering from which we often hide by use of our innumerable accessories of distraction. Vulnerable, raw and unflinching, our guide looks death square in the face. But always with effective, practical reflections that are saturated with wisdom and our author's growing awareness of the presence and lovingkindness of the God who in Jesus suffers with us. For those who long to know that they are not alone in the confusion that suffering and death bring, this is a trustworthy place to start.

Curt Thompson, MD, author of *The Soul of Desire* **and** *The Deepest Place: Suffering and the Formation of Hope*

There are few times when life's big questions hang in the balance so profoundly as when you walk with someone to the line between life on earth and life beyond. Through his account of his wife Heather's diagnosis, treatment, and death, Bob Cutillo captures the process as a husband and physician, with candor and grace.

There are also few times in life when someone is able to recount with depth a shared profound experience. I also witnessed this holy process, because Heather was my friend and mentor. The book holds the tension of pain and beauty that is the profound essence of life moving toward death. When Heather was diagnosed with cancer I was certain God would protect his faithful servant, and yet she reminded me she did not have a special exception from suffering. Bob does the same, offering the reader a biblical paradigm for life, death, and grief.

For the reader who is wondering why a loving God allows faithful people to suffer, this book will be your companion. Bob's life as a physician has positioned him to understand sickness and death with a clinical lens. His role as a husband and caretaker provides an overlay to that head knowledge with reflections of the heart and heartbreak to these same themes. Far from sterile, you will find tender, thoughtful honesty that surrenders to God's good will for both the patient and the caretaker, the loved and the one left to grieve.

This is a must read for anyone who dares to live by daring to love.

Alexandra Kuykendall, author of *Seeking Out Goodness: Finding the True and Beautiful all Around You*

Holding on in the Storm is a deeply valuable text for anyone caught in the vortex of suffering. The book will be helpful for ministry professionals, such as chaplains, pastors, and ministers, who frequently have one hand holding Jesus while the other hand grasps the suffering. Cutillo clearly encourages the paramount importance of Christian belief and consistently exemplifies faith throughout the book. He vividly uses Scripture that connects the reader to various emotions of suffering. Rarely does any author write with both the width of experience and depth of loss as Cutillo. His book touches the reader with compassion, offering tools for pastoral ministry and spiritual care "for the least, the lost, and the left out."

Cutillo reminds us of spiritual tools that are provided by God, undergirded by the Bible, which embolden us to face our vulnerability to sickness, suffering, and death as creatures in a fallen world. In the end, as it was at the beginning, Cutillo reminds us of Jesus' true purpose in John 16:33, "But take heart; I have overcome the world."

Alan T. "Blues" Baker, Supervisor of Chaplain Ministries, Reformed Church in America, and author of *Foundations of Chaplaincy: A Practical Guide*

I have known Dr. Bob Cutillo since he came to work at Lawndale Christian Health Center in 1984, where he also met his wife, Heather. I remember them falling in love and had the privilege to co-officiate their wedding with Heather's father. I have considered Bob a good friend ever since, and I have watched his life and ministry with admiration after he left Lawndale. From the beginning he has been a man of integrity, deeply committed to Christ, and tireless in caring for people—especially those on the margins.

What I love about this book is how Bob reminds us that medicine is not simply a science to master, but a gift to receive, a care to extend, and a way to honor the dignity of every human life. He challenges our assumptions, inviting us to move beyond control and cure to the deeper work of compassion and presence. These words reflect not only his convictions but also the way he has lived for over forty years.

I wholeheartedly recommend this book. It offers wisdom, hope, and a vision of health and healing that our world desperately needs today.

Wayne "Coach" Gordon, Pastor Emeritus, Lawndale Community Church, Professor, Northern Seminary

Holding on in the Storm

Biblical wisdom for courage
and guidance through sickness,
suffering, death, and grief

Bob Cutillo, MD

For more information and a free discussion guide, visit:

HoldingOnInTheStorm.com

Scripture quotations are from the ESV® Bible (The Holy Bible, English Standard Version®), © 2001 by Crossway, a publishing ministry of Good News Publishers. Used by permission. All rights reserved. The ESV text may not be quoted in any publication made available to the public by a Creative Commons license. The ESV may not be translated in whole or in part into any other language.

Copyright © 2025 by Bob Cutillo, MD
All Rights Reserved
ISBN: 978-1-64180-232-1
Version 1.0

Cover design by Rick Nease
RickNeaseArt.com

Author photo by Jamie Ringoen

Published by Read the Spirit Books
42807 Ford Road
No. 234
Canton, MI, 48187

Front Edge Publishing books are available for discount bulk purchases for events, corporate use and small groups. Special editions, including books with corporate logos, personalized covers and customized interiors are available for purchase. For more information, contact Front Edge Publishing at info@FrontEdgePublishing.com.

Contents

About the Cover xvi
Foreword by Kate Miller xvii
Author's Introduction xxii

Chapter 1: Meeting Heather 1
Chapter 2: The Test Result 10
Chapter 3: The Diagnosis 16
Chapter 4: Treatment Begins 27
Chapter 5: A Good Response to Treatment 36
Chapter 6: Another Encounter With Death 46
Chapter 7: The End of Treatment 57
Chapter 8: Crossing Over 70
Chapter 9: A Mystical Union 83
Chapter 10: Stunned 92
Chapter 11: A Thought That Had to Change 102
Chapter 12: Collecting Scattered Pieces 110
Chapter 13: How Long, O Lord? 126
Chapter 14: Embracing God's *Chesed* 137

Finding Solace in Scripture 146
Additional Support and Further Reading 154
Acknowledgments 156
About the Author 160

To Heather, my cherished wife,
"A tree planted by streams of water, that yields its fruit in its season, and its leaf does not wither."
Psalm 1:3

About the Cover

When I first saw Rembrandt's painting, *A Storm on the Sea of Galilee*, many years ago, I was intrigued by the capacity of this painting to draw me so intimately into this Scriptural passage. The Gospels of Matthew, Mark, and Luke (Matthew 8:23-27, Mark 4:35-41, Luke 8: 22-25) all contain this beautiful but brief story of Jesus getting into a boat on a quiet day. But then sometime after the journey begins, without warning, a furious storm appears, putting all in the boat in grave danger. In the painting we see the urgency and terror as several of the disciples desperately try to hang on and keep the boat from capsizing.

A key component of this story is that Jesus is asleep in the stern—until the terrified disciples wake him up. "Teacher, don't you care?" they cry out. "Lord, save us, we are going to drown."

I find many connections to my journey with my wife, Heather, after she was diagnosed with terminal cancer—a storm that came out of nowhere, sending me reeling and reaching to hold on for dear life. There were times when I wondered if Jesus was asleep. "Lord, don't you care?" I would cry out. "I feel like I am drowning. Save me!"

But please look closely at this painting for a detail I find utterly fascinating. As you look carefully into all the corners of the ship, you see that there are fourteen people in the boat. Yes, it is true. Besides Jesus and the twelve, Rembrandt has put himself in the story. There he is, in the middle of the boat, looking bewildered with his hand on his head, staring directly at the viewer.

I always admired this painting for this personal addition. For in the strokes of his brush that place him in the picture, I believe he is telling us that the most fruitful way to read Scripture is to put yourself in the story.

For many years, I tried to follow that advice. And then my wife got very sick and eventually died. I no longer had to try to put myself in the story. The sickness, suffering, and death of my wife put me in that boat whether I wanted it or not. The storms of life have a way of forcing us into places that are not of our own choosing. Suddenly we are in the midst of a raging storm, and we are deathly afraid. And with us is Jesus, who is not in the least overwhelmed by the circumstances. On his command the waves roll back, the storm subsides, and the sea becomes completely calm.

And then Jesus turns to us with a question, one that echoes through the centuries for each of us to ponder in every age: "Why are you so afraid, O you of little faith?"

Bob Cutillo

Care to look more deeply into this painting? Follow this QR code to see a much higher-resolution version.

Foreword

To those who knew me growing up, it may have come as a surprise that I ended up choosing the same career path as my mother, becoming a pediatric nurse practitioner. Or maybe not. Most of my friends recognized what special people my parents were, and the very close relationship we shared with one another. To follow in their footsteps was an honor. In late high school and college, I vowed I wouldn't go into medicine "just because my parents did." And yet I ended up understanding what they had instilled in me—a life devoted to caring for others was a gift, a beautiful opportunity to be welcomed into others' lives through the vulnerability shared in health and sickness. When cancer brought that vulnerability directly into my own family, it was undoubtedly one of the most heart-wrenching times in my life. I also consider it an immense privilege to have walked with my parents on their journey. Through my dad's intimate retelling in this book of the last few years of my mom's life, and the grief that followed after her death, I hope and pray that as the reader you will get to share in that beautiful experience as well.

At work recently I was brought back to a fear that many people in health care experience. A young woman was worried that the rash she had for several weeks must be life-threatening since it wasn't going away. The rash was benign, but it viscerally brought me back to the days when I was studying for my master's and was crippled by anxiety that I or someone close to me might suffer from the terrible diseases I was reading about. I distinctly remember looking at the predisposing risks for each cancer, and then trying to assuage my fears by convincing myself that those awful things couldn't happen to me or my family because none of us had those risk factors. For me, a diagnosis of incurable cancer was one of the worst things I could imagine.

Many years later, my mother was diagnosed with one of my worst fears. After processing my initial shock, I soon saw that despite my fears of being abandoned to suffering and grief, the actuality was much less terrifying than the possibility. I immediately felt that God was with us. I found that God made himself available to us in a more intimate way than maybe most of us have ever experienced. My prayer throughout the years of cancer treatment and ultimately my mother's death was that I would know God's presence and peace in the midst of suffering. And God was so near when we needed him most.

Almost four months before she died, I was on a walk in my neighborhood, listening to worship music, when I had a profound sense that my mom didn't have long to live. The lyrics specifically described a person sitting by a woman's hospital bed, but trusting that God was still worthy. I had listened to the song many times before, but this time it stood out, like flashing lights on a neon sign. At that time in her treatment, there was a clinical trial her doctors were considering, and so as a family we were hopeful that she would qualify and it could give us more time together. In that moment, I remember being fearful of what then this "sense" meant: What did it mean that I felt like God was preparing me for the end? Could I still hope that the trial might be something helpful to her? As I listened to the same song on repeat, praying and crying out to God, I felt like he was giving me the opportunity to grieve then, in that moment, because he was preparing me for what was to come. There was no indication as to "when," just that God would not leave us throughout any of it. I was being asked to be strong, stay steadfast, and know that I would not be alone.

From that time of preparation several months before my mom passed away, I was given a strength that was very much outside of myself. And it was very clear that it was a gift, that God had prepared me and he would stay with all of us. I saw the same in my parents—a steadiness and peace that transcended all understanding. Each decision was made, not in anxiety or fear, but from a deep sense that God was over and in everything. The last big decision they made was to not enroll in the clinical trial that was the final option available. Their wise oncologist did not give them false hope, and ultimately advised against it as it was likely to cause more pain with very little healing. As I watched my parents accept this reality, I saw them do so without hesitation because they felt that God was over all of their decisions.

My mom had one last hospital visit about two months before she died, when yet another bowel obstruction brought her to seek care. I spent many hours with her during this hospitalization, much more than before when visitation restrictions were in place due to the COVID pandemic.

My mom remained the caregiver in the room despite being the one at the center of needing care. She encouraged a new nurse practicing her first nasogastric tube, "Oh, back when I was in school we had to practice on each other!" She asked about her life. How was her new job going? She even encouraged me as I sat with her, telling me what a good support I was for her. And when the things they tried in the hospital failed and she was being discharged home to begin hospice care, she only told me after asking how the day had gone for my kids at school. Always focused on others, my family and the people my mom encountered were blessed by her loving heart. She modeled truly being the hands and feet of Jesus to everyone she met.

I hope that, through this book, you will see what I saw throughout my whole life, and most poignantly in the last several years of my mom's life—that life with Jesus is not always an easy life, but it is undoubtedly a good life. My parents' love for one another and their deep faith and trust in an unwavering God allowed them to walk through a gut-wrenching time of suffering with hope, trusting that God was with them. And while one would never hope for suffering, we were met with an intimacy with Jesus that was unlike any I had experienced before, a kindness he extended to us in our suffering, and an acute awareness of his loving and compassionate nature.

May you see God's care for your grief, your suffering, and your burdens as you read the experience of my dad as he said goodbye to the love of his life, held by a God who cares so deeply for our hurting hearts.

Kate Miller is Bob and Heather's daughter. She is a pediatric nurse practitioner who lives in Colorado.

Author's Introduction

*Any man's death diminishes me, because I am involved in Mankind;
And therefore never send to know for whom the bell tolls;
it tolls for thee.*

John Donne

Sickness, loss, and death often are thrust upon us without warning—but I believe that, out of those moments when life breaks into pieces, new purpose can arise.

Many of us walk through the world each day barely perceiving that there is only one source of goodness—and it is God. But if our world explodes with the loss of the most precious person we know, all previous certainties seem to fall away. We stop, stunned, and realize there is nothing of value apart from God. So, we run to God and cling to God with all the might we can muster.

And then we discover that God has been holding onto us since the day we were born.

In 2016, I wrote a book from a place of deep concern for the pain of others. Based on my experiences as a physician caring for the disenfranchised, I tried to help readers see the world through their eyes. I sought to offer a redeemed view of health that would care for all. At the same time, I hoped that my book would better prepare readers to face the inevitabilities of sickness and death when they arrived. I hoped it would better prepare me for my own journey when I faced sickness and death.

I did not realize then how much harder my test would be. This current book is a story of sadness, grief, and grace, when health is lost, and death is imminent. Not my loss of health, or my fear of death, but far worse, the loss of health and the death of my wife. All that I believed was true when I wrote *Pursuing Health in an Anxious Age* was thoroughly tried by our journey together through my wife's incurable cancer.

Suddenly, I was living through the challenges I had tried to confidently explain in *Pursuing Health*. A major theme of that first book was that health is a gift from God and not a possession. Now I was being asked to apply that same truth in my relationship with my wife. If ever I thought she belonged to me, I was sadly mistaken. Given to me, but never mine to possess. As are all the greatest treasures in life, they come as a gift undeserved, given by the giver of all good things. As James reminds us, "Every good gift and every perfect gift is from above, coming down from the Father of Lights" (James 1:17). This is the lesson I had to learn at the most intimate level. Living through this journey—the long and arduous course of Heather's cancer and death—I found my own world rocked. I was humbled. I found myself struggling and learning at a greater spiritual depth than I had ever experienced in my life as a physician.

This book is a testimony of my particular journey. I am offering my story in the hope that you will find some of your own story in these pages, whether you have lost a precious person, place, career—or dream. Maybe your journey is a decline in health that you cannot reclaim. And now you are being asked to let it go, lest you try to hold on to what you cannot keep. Rather than a teacher offering a lesson or an expert making a presentation, I am writing in these pages as one friend telling his story to another—and asking for prayer.

This book is my effort to attest to the truth that God, the giver of all good things, is always good and more than worthy of our trust.

The format of this book opens with medical milestones familiar to millions, starting with testing, diagnosis, and treatment. If you have encountered poet John Donne's classic meditations on illness, death, and rebirth, called *Devotions Upon Emergent Occasions*, then you may recognize some of the basic rhythms as this book unfolds. Donne documented the step-by-step progress of his life-threatening illness and the reflections he had in response to the stage of disease he was experiencing. Following his pattern, each of my chapters includes a narrative account of a stage on the journey of sickness, death, and grief, then a section on "Challenges to biblical faith" related to that stage, followed by a reflection that draws strength from a specific biblical passage.

Early on, Heather started to write about her experiences under the tentative title, "The Journey of My Abdominal Pain." I quote from her writings early in this book. But, much to our loss, she did not continue journaling. Too many things got in the way. Sickness and reactions to chemotherapy on the negative side—and, on the positive side, her outgoing spirit led her, when feeling well, to spend most of her time caring for others rather than writing about her own condition. Fortunately, Heather did make time to write on her CaringBridge webpage to keep friends and family aware of how she was doing. It will be part of my attempt in this book to use those rich resources, plus my own intimate memories.

By its very nature, this account of our journey together—and my own experiences beyond her death—is my own. I am sharing it, not to glorify our story, but because the remembrance of our story and the retelling of that story may help someone like you to find the resilience you need to travel just a little further yourself.

And in that goal of helping others, I know that Heather shares in this adventure.

1

Meeting Heather

*Do not be conformed to this world,
but be transformed by the renewal of your mind,
that by testing you may discern what is the will of God,
what is good and acceptable and perfect.*

Romans 12:2

My first date with Heather began as an emergency.

The phone call on a July evening in 1985 was not unexpected, yet still disorienting as Heather awoke from a sound sleep. It was her new friend Sandra, and she was in labor. Heather had made a commitment six months earlier to be with Sandra for all her prenatal visits and then coach her through her labor and delivery. It was time to honor her promise. But first she had to call me and let me know the news. That's because I was Sandra's doctor.

Heather at the time was in her master's level training to be a pediatric nurse practitioner. She was also in a Bible study with fellow nurses who as a group decided to volunteer at Lawndale Christian Health Center on the west side of Chicago. The clinic had just opened a few months earlier and was committed to making good health care accessible to an underserved community. I had just finished my residency in family practice at Cook County Hospital and joined the initial group of three doctors to start the clinic.

When Heather asked the medical director if she could follow a woman through her pregnancy and delivery as part of her training, he told her the only doctor who delivered babies was me.

How serendipitous in so many ways! I knew someone who could really use her help. Sandra had suffered a great deal of trauma and abuse in her life, and besides being poor and without family, she was now pregnant with little support. Having Heather to walk with her through this pregnancy was just what Sandra needed. From this chance encounter, Sandra and I gained far more than we could have ever asked or imagined.

Of course, Heather did what Heather always did. She learned about Sandra's life, experienced deep empathy for the pain and abuse that Sandra had suffered, and committed to caring for her through the pregnancy and beyond. She became her friend and gained her trust by treating her with dignity and respect, offering Sandra a kind of trusting relationship she had rarely experienced.

The night of the delivery turned out to be an all-night affair. Heather was with Sandra throughout the labor, and I arrived as labor progressed toward what we hoped would be a normal delivery. But, to put it simply, the baby got stuck. In medical jargon, it was a "failure to progress." We had to call the obstetrician who came and performed a cesarean section. Heather was with Sandra through it all, and instead of delivering the baby myself my role became caring for the newborn.

As this long and sleepless night unfolded—we eventually realized the sun was coming up!

We all were exhausted. And hungry.

"Feel like breakfast?" I asked.

"Sure," Heather said.

The setup for that first date was as simple as that—a shared need for coffee and something to eat after a harrowing night coupled with our mutual desire to linger just a little longer in the warm aura of gratefulness we felt over helping to assist with a healthy birth.

We drove a few miles west to a Greek diner that has been a local landmark in the town of Berwyn. Even if you've never seen it, you know the place: Formica tables, plastic-covered menus that could easily be wiped down, and so many choices that it boggled the mind how one little kitchen could make that many different things.

We spoke little—at least nothing I can remember now after all these years.

We did not need to say much, because we shared such a profound experience of helping Sandra—against all the tough odds in her life—to bring her child into the world.

I will never forget that, even before our food arrived, we prayed. Simply. Spontaneously. We poured out our thankfulness for the opportunities God had given us to provide care through that little Christian clinic. And we voiced our thanks for all of the people of faith who had made that clinic possible and had truly surrounded Sandra with a life-giving presence at the start of her baby's life.

We could feel God's grace surrounding us in that little diner.

Between our first breakfast together and the one we shared at that same diner eight months later, on the morning of our wedding, I came to learn a great deal more about

Heather. I came to appreciate how deeply she cared about the mission of God in a broken and hurting world.

Heather was brought up in a pastor's home and, unlike some pastors' kids, she loved being at church multiple times every week and doing all the things that the other kids in her youth group did. Because her father was the head of an international mission program, she met many missionaries when they came to speak at her church. Early in life, when she was only nine years old, she made a commitment to serve God with her life. This commitment was reinforced through her confirmation class at age twelve, when she was baptized. At the time she chose Romans 12:1-2 as her life verses:

> I appeal to you therefore, brothers and sisters, by the mercies of God, to present your bodies as a living sacrifice, holy and acceptable to God, which is your spiritual worship. Do not be conformed to this world, but be transformed by the renewal of your mind, that by testing you may discern what is the will of God, what is good and acceptable and perfect.

She wanted to follow Jesus with her whole heart.

What I also learned about Heather in those eight months before our marriage was how much fun she was. That was good because I can be a bit on the serious side. On my birthday in August, she cooked up a plan with our friends to kidnap me, blindfold me, put me in the trunk of a car, and take me to some unknown destination for a birthday party. I had no idea what a ride I was in for, both that day and for the rest of our lives together.

Meeting Heather

Heather had a glad heart and a cheerful face—like a vision right out of Proverbs 15:13. Her face broke into a smile more easily than anyone I knew, a sweet smile accompanied by joyful and twinkling eyes. Her bright countenance made others feel welcome and comfortable in her presence. I suppose that is why so many people found it so easy to talk with her. This also made her a good mentor. Early in our marriage she committed to mentoring two teenage girls in our inner-city church, Eunice and Theresa. She poured herself into their lives, encouraging them in their walk of faith and their prayer life. To this day Eunice is a close friend of our family who has lived faithfully and has passed on that heritage to her two sons with the strong support of her loving husband.

While Heather and I were serving in urban mission at the clinic and church in Lawndale, we wondered if God might be calling us beyond the United States to another country. I had been entertaining that idea since first becoming a doctor, but Heather was far beyond me. She had already served for two years as a missionary nurse in a rural hospital in Mukinge in the northwest corner of Zambia. Out in such isolated places, her work had expanded dramatically—simply because there was no one else out there who could help. She delivered babies, sutured wounds, cared for patients with tuberculosis and leprosy, and trained local nurses.

There were two highlights of these years that Heather always mentioned. One was the Bible study she had with ten student nurses over two years where she got to know them as individuals and encourage their faith. The other notable memory was a relationship she developed with a woman in a neighboring village who had leprosy. Her name was Kapa

Baya. Heather rode a motorcycle back then and she would drive to this village for church and then stay afterward at Kapa Baya's house. "She was my grandma," she said, a joyful and godly woman who she remembered for the rest of her life.

With much deliberation, after four years at Lawndale, we did accept a call to be missionaries to Zaire, now the Democratic Republic of Congo. Remaining committed to urban mission, we were sent to help the local church begin a primary care clinic in the capital city of Kinshasa. It was a turbulent time in a country that had suffered and would continue to suffer through many turbulent times. In this case it was due to a corrupt and greedy government led by President Mobutu, at the time one of the richest men in the world while leading one of the poorest countries. In the midst of extreme hyperinflation, the military was paid with paper money that held its value for less than a day. Our time in Kinshasa ended abruptly on September 23, 1991, when the military revolted. The city was ransacked, tanks rolled in the streets. After three days of chaos, the United States called for an evacuation of all of its citizens. Quickly ferried across the Congo River to Brazzaville, the capital of the neighboring Republic of Congo, we flew on a government-chartered flight back to the United States. Allowed only one bag per person, we left many things behind. But there were two things we refused to leave: family photos, of course, but also Legos. For our two-year-old and four-year-old children, Legos were everything. Who needs dishes and towels!

After the evacuation, we looked stateside for other mission opportunities. It was always in our minds that God had brought us together for a purpose. Our marriage was "made in Lawndale," as our former pastor used to say, and its birth within a mission setting only solidified our individual calls to mission.

Heather and I were a unique blend. I think only God could have seen how well we would bond together, making something round and something square somehow fit. I will never forget the comment of the psychologist who interviewed and tested us to assess our qualities and capabilities for being cross-cultural missionaries. At the end of two days of grueling questioning, his summary comment was, "I have never seen a couple so different who are such a good match."

One of Heather's greatest attributes was her flexibility and adaptability. We ended up doing health care work in mission contexts in numerous locations over the years. In Washington, D.C., we worked with the homeless and underserved at Christ House and Columbia Road Health Services. Heather was mostly a mother to our young children, Kate and Steve, but also worked two times a week in the health center. A special memory of this time was getting to meet Mother Teresa. One day she came to the health center to thank the staff. It was our clinic that provided medical care to the orphans cared for by her Missionaries of Charity and Heather was their primary practitioner. She especially enjoyed these visits because of the love these children received from the sisters.

We were recommissioned to go back to Zaire in 1998, but just before we arrived the country fell into a civil war. We were sent to South Africa to wait and see what would happen. Heather adapted to the change and joined other missionary families in forming a home school for all the children. Unfortunately, the war continued, and we were never able to safely enter the country.

In our years in Denver, we worked at another Christian clinic, Inner City Health Center. They didn't really need Heather's pediatric skills, but they needed a certified diabetes educator. Once again Heather reprogrammed herself and got the training to meet the need. Later, she joined a friend who wanted to start a school for pregnant and parenting teens with day care for their children. They needed a school nurse. As usual, Heather changed course, got the necessary certifications, and became the child and student health coordinator for New Legacy Charter School.

Heather's flexibility and adaptability allowed her to share in the lives of many people. She had a way of crossing boundaries and offering unbiased love to those who had suffered a lack of enduring love before. She always felt that God especially cared for the afflicted and poor, and the commitment she had made long before to offer herself as a "living sacrifice" meant caring for the least, the lost, and the left out.

But there was one thing Heather did not like to share. I learned about it early in our engagement and almost ruined it. After a movie, we decided to go for an ice cream cone. I suggested we buy a double-dip and share it, and we could save some money. The look on her face was stern and firm. Each one of us would have our own ice cream cone. There was no debate. An ice cream cone is something you don't share.

Perhaps the one word that most defines who Heather was is "caregiver." Whether caring for our children, caring for the children in her pediatric practice, or mentoring moms at MOPS International and caring for their children—she was the ultimate caregiver. Many of our children's friends wanted to come over to our house because of the way Heather cared about them. She devotedly cared for her parents after her father had a devastating stroke that left him severely disabled for the last ten years of his life.

She had always embraced this role as her primary purpose in life. I think that is why she assumed that we would grow old together and one day she would care for me. But that is not how it turned out.

We did not grow old together.

Much to our surprise, she was the one who would need the care, and I was the one who would give it.

2

The Test Result

*God whispers to us in our pleasures,
speaking in our conscience,
but shouts in our pains:
It is God's megaphone to rouse a deaf world.*

C.S. Lewis

The phone call on Tuesday evening, March 24, 2020, though not awakening us from sleep, was far more disorienting than Sandra's phone calls to us thirty-five years earlier. This call was from our primary care physician, Dr. Edward Ho. Heather's ongoing stomach pains had prompted a visit to Dr. Ho, who ordered a CT scan.

Now, he was calling with the results—and they were ominous.

"I wanted to get back to you as soon as I got these results," he told us as he delivered the news, knowing he was talking to health care professionals. "The report suggests there is some tumor growing around Heather's stomach and it seems to have spread to other parts of her abdomen."

Heather remained silent, listening intently.

"It sounds serious, Ed," I remember saying.

He tried to soften the blow, reaching for several possibilities that offered less dangerous and life-threatening outcomes. But we knew in our hearts that malignant cancer was most likely. As he described the tumor, it appeared to be so thickly matted together that it was beginning to distort and twist the intestines. An exploratory abdominal surgery with biopsy was needed to confirm a diagnosis.

The next day I was scheduled to see patients at a Colorado Coalition for the Homeless clinic in Denver, where I worked. At that time COVID cases were sharply on the rise. This sickness—unknown and frightful as it first surfaced—was mostly confined to China in January 2020, but by March had quickly spread throughout the world. On January 31, the World Health Organization (WHO) had declared it a global health emergency. By March 11, COVID was declared a pandemic. On March 13, with growing spread into the United States, the president declared it a national emergency. Health care institutions throughout the United States, upended by this sudden turn of events, scrambled to come up with safety protocols that would reduce the transmission of the disease. We were especially concerned about the protection of ourselves and our colleagues as we tried to provide ongoing health care.

At that time, Heather and I knew so little about the weight, the length, and the depth of the journey we were about to begin! However, sometime during that Tuesday night—between getting the phone call from Dr. Ho and the time of my next shift—I realized that I could not return to work. I was concerned about the unknowns of COVID as a contagious and life-threatening illness and its potential impact on the unknowns of my wife's current condition, especially if she had to undergo chemotherapy.

Already, that night was forever changing our lives. It felt as if one moment was light—and now dark surrounded us.

As professionals, we both had seen bad things happen in our patients' lives, so it wasn't as if we thought this could never happen to us or to one of our loved ones. Still, the shock of this news in our own lives was disorienting. We had counseled others and prayed for them, but now our faith was under trial.

Would our faith remain an anchor? Or would the looming storms rage until our anchor was torn loose?

Challenges to biblical faith

Our culture poorly prepares us to receive bad news. Most of us assume bad things happen elsewhere and to other people. Wars and floods happen in other countries. There are murders and drug overdoses, but they happen in other neighborhoods. And fatal illnesses? They happen in other families.

For years, we have nourished a false sense of security and invulnerability with a steady diet of quick fixes for every problem. We have fueled a fantasy that we are in control of life. As I wrote previously, "Somehow the idea that life can be controlled to our satisfaction by a mixture of good behavior, good choices, good medicine, or a good God—if God does what we expect—enters into the pores of our being without our notice."

By some trick of our imagination, we have forgotten that this world is a risky and often hostile place. We have buffered ourselves for so long that, when bad news comes, not only are we thoroughly frightened by it, but also completely inexperienced in how to trust God with it. In the moment of a sudden change in our circumstances, our first hope is not in God, but in the medical technology that will fix what broke. Harking back to an analogy I used in *Pursuing Health in an Anxious Age*, we are like Humpty Dumpty. Though we sit on a precarious wall in our fragile shells, we are oblivious to any mortal danger—until we fall. And when we do, like Humpty, we are certain that "all the king's army and all the king's men" will find a way to put us back together again.

But what if that doesn't happen?

Turning to the Bible

*It is well with the man who deals generously and
lends; who conducts his affairs with justice.
For the righteous will never be moved,
he will be remembered forever.
He is not afraid of bad news;
his heart is firm, trusting in the Lord. …
He has distributed freely;
he has given to the poor;
his righteousness endures forever;
his horn is exalted in honor.*

From Psalm 112

Wouldn't we all like to be this person when bad news comes? That's who I wanted to be on that night of Dr. Ho's call—but we never know for sure if we have measured up. I wondered: Have I been as generous in my life as this man in Psalm 112? Have I conducted my affairs with a true concern for justice that makes me like him?

But all those uncertainties just revealed my confusion. This ideal figure in Psalm 112 is not secure *because* he did these things. He *did these things* because he trusted in God. His trust in God is what makes him secure. And that made my questions more piercing and to the point: Can God be trusted? Could I trust God now with my wife's life?

Whenever life is interrupted by some tragic or difficult circumstance, this is the basic issue we face. Whether it takes the form of a phone call with a dreaded test result, or an email telling us we are being laid off, or a son telling us he is divorcing his wife—in each case, our world seems to turn upside down. The world we thought we controlled is shifting around us.

In every traumatic case, the same questions need answers: Is God good? Can God be trusted to keep the promises we read in the Bible?

And that is what we *tried* to do from the first night—trust God. But the road was far more twisted, and the level of sadness and loss much more profound than we could have ever anticipated.

We were not yet ready to see how hard the work of faith would be if our anchor was to hold.

For reflection and discussion

1. When was the last time your world was turned upside down by news of a sad and unexpected event? How did you react?

2. When bad things happen in your life, do you assume it is your fault? Or do you blame others? Or do you turn your anger toward God for allowing it to happen?

3. Does the model of the psalmist help you to better prepare to receive bad news?

3

The Diagnosis

*Midway along the journey of my life,
I woke to find myself in a dark wood.*

Dante

On April 1, 2020, a little over a week after Dr. Ho phoned with the results of the CT scan, Heather had exploratory surgery.

Mercifully, we had reached that point in a short time. There was urgency in the air given how quickly Heather's health was failing. Each day the advance of intestinal blockages was weakening her ability to eat and maintain her strength. Any delay in diagnosis might make it too late for an effective treatment. We saw the surgeon on March 31. Given the gravity of the situation, he scheduled the operation for the very next day. If there was any silver lining to the early onset of the storm of COVID coming at the same time as the cancer, it was that no elective surgeries were being scheduled, leaving the operating room schedule wide open.

When the surgeon came to the waiting room on that Wednesday afternoon to explain what he had found, I tried to be ready to hear the worst. And the worst was what it was. Heather had an aggressively growing cancer scattered throughout her abdomen. The pathology results a few days later confirmed what was already suspected—an incurable advanced stage 4 gastric cancer with a very limited prognosis. The most practical question in that hour was if Heather's deteriorating physical condition would be able to tolerate the toxic chemotherapy that had the potential to shrink the tumor.

In these early days of pursuing a diagnosis, our reactions were difficult to control. Whatever we might encounter, we knew it would test us like never before. It was important to pull back from panic mode whenever the pendulum of emotions swung in that direction. We wanted to be in a place where we could take the needed steps without looking too far down the road. Of course, we wanted to continue as long as possible, so we needed a way to walk together on this road fraught with overwhelming fears. We had to find a way of sustaining our hope.

We needed companions and I found one kindred spirit in Dante Alighieri, the famous Italian poet. His poignant search for eternal truth grounded in the common realities of everyday life always reminded me that God is near and dear in the ups and downs of life. In his masterpiece, *The Divine Comedy*, Dante writes about himself as a pilgrim setting out on a journey of growth. He calls it a path from bondage to freedom.

This is everyone's journey when we feel lost and need to recover the true path. I am certainly not alone in this. Bob Dylan sensed it, too, as he describes in *Tangled Up in Blue*. In the midst of despair, Dylan sings that a woman—out of the blue—asked him to read Dante. As he did:

> Every one of them words rang true
> And glowed like burnin' coal
> Pourin' off of every page
> Like it was written in my soul from me to you

Like Dylan, I commend Dante's treasure trove to you, because of his solid faith that this lost wanderer will find his way home. That's in spite of the fact that Dante's metaphorical journey begins in a very dark place:

> Midway along the journey of our life, I woke to find myself in a dark wood, for I had wandered off from the straight path. How hard it is to tell what it is like, this wood of wilderness, savage and stubborn—the thought of it brings back all my old fears. A bitter place! Death could scarce be bitterer. But if I would show the good that came of it, I must talk about things other than the good. How I entered there I cannot truly say.

These truths ring universally, whether you're Dante or Dylan or the two of us reeling from such lifechanging news. Neither Heather nor I could explain how or why we had entered our own dark wood. Just a few days before, the sun was high in the sky. We never saw the dark clouds coming.

Six days before the surgery, Heather had enough energy to write down some of her thoughts and feelings as she heroically stepped into this dark wood with me:

> It could be very bad. My current hope is that it's some parasite I picked up in Africa which is causing havoc but can be treated. That would be amazing! Of course, knowing this could be very

> serious is very sobering—my thoughts go all over the place. ... I do have a sense of peace that God knows all this already and that He is with me whatever happens. ... Metastatic cancer doesn't sound good. I realized maybe part of the reason I can't wrap my head around this is that usually I am the caregiver. I'm a nurse, a mom, a grandma. I cared for my dad so many years, and mom. It's weird to be the one who is going to need help. I guess if I ever thought about it in my head, I would have thought I'd be the one caring for Bob in our old age. I guess I have some things to learn. How can I do this? How can I live into this and learn more about God's love and my dependence on Him? How can I help bless others during this time?

Three days before the surgery, she wrote:

> Today is Sunday—the readings were all about the resurrection. God breathing life into dry bones in Ezekiel, Lazarus raised from the dead, Martha, who "got" who Jesus was. Despite her flaws of trying too hard, Jesus loved her, helped her understand, and she *got it* and trusted Him. May I be like that. Then Romans 8—the Spirit of Life sets me free from the law of sin and death. His Spirit in me—LIFE through him in me. And back to Lazarus: "This sickness will not end in death. No, it is for God's glory, so that God's Son may be glorified through it" (John 11:4). Lord, I don't know where this is going but I pray you will

help me trust you and Lord, may you be glorified in it.

Heather was expressing so much wisdom, even though she knew hardly anything about what was to come. Yes, Heather entertained a small hope it was something infectious from her missionary days in Africa. But when she looked up and saw the darkness around her, the thought of metastatic cancer was overwhelming. Already she anticipated changing roles, ones she never thought she would occupy. I would be the primary caregiver on this journey for one who was the most excellent of caregivers.

Would I be up to that task?

How beautiful to see these Scriptures Heather had in hand as she was about to step forward on this path. She saw a Savior who is the resurrection and the life, who assures us that "whoever believes in me, though he die, yet shall he live, and everyone who lives and believes in me shall never die. Do you believe this?" (John 11: 25-26).

Martha *got it*, and Heather wanted to *get it* too. Already she was preparing to face the unknown with a hope in the resurrection. And she desired to grow in her love and dependence on God so that she could be a blessing to others.

But if we "would show the good," as Dante desired on his journey, we too "must talk about things other than the good." And that is where we will go next.

Challenges to biblical faith

I could not help it. I had to read up on Heather's cancer. And after looking up medical references on the prognosis for stage 4 gastric cancer, the number six kept coming up. An average time of survival of six months. To some extent such sobering information might be helpful. But what did that mean for Heather?

Heather was not a statistic! Heather was a particular person with gastric cancer.

Given how aggressively the cancer was moving without treatment, she could easily die much sooner. But what if the treatment took hold? What if other treatments became available? What if God intended some miraculous work?

In *Pursuing Health in an Anxious Age*, I described how probability and statistics in medicine become a disembodied way of looking at patients and their future prognosis. I wrote, "Increasingly, medical science is approving only one source of knowledge, that which is 'proven' by statistics. If something is cloaked in numbers, it must be true. But incomplete data, multiple sources of bias, and bewildering complexity producing results of implausible precision are making it difficult to determine when the results are valid and, more importantly, when the outcomes are meaningful for our individual lives."

The ability to predict the outcome of disease has always been an important function in medicine. The father of Western medicine, Hippocrates, considered it an essential function. He wrote: "It appears to me a most excellent thing for the physician to cultivate Prognosis; for by foreseeing and foretelling, in the presence of the sick, the present, the past, and the future ... he will be the more readily believed to be acquainted with the circumstances of the sick; so that men will have confidence to entrust themselves to such a physician."

Without the benefit of statistical models, he taught his protégés to master the art of prognostication by observing the patient with the utmost interest and concentration, focusing on details such as the position of the body, the movement of the hands, and the expressions of the face. Nowadays, the tools and technology of our age have pushed aside such observations in favor of numbers and averages.

As I wrote in *Pursuing Health*, "Today, we still prognosticate but usually with a much different approach, less likely to observe the patient and far more inclined to look at survival statistics or disease progression likelihoods. In one sense this is more accurate. Having data to show what has happened to people with disease X, we can calculate the average survival, and even perhaps estimate how existing treatments can alter the outcome. Patients currently with disease X can look at these numbers as a way to predict what will happen to them."

But what do they see, hear, and internalize when a health care professional gives them these numbers? And, more importantly, can these statistics answer their most important questions? Whatever the statistics show, no one is just an average. Deep down we know we are more than an abstraction. For each one, there is no percentage or probability but only a particular path.

Interestingly, our oncologists rarely brought up the numbers as we talked. I think they knew the information was dismal—so what was the use of flattening our hopes with these statistical hammers? Perhaps they would have taken a different tack if Heather or I were overly optimistic to the point of having unrealistic expectations of what treatment could do. But our spirit of engagement with this news was rooted in a hope that God was in control, a belief that treatment could offer some good, and a desire to begin as soon as possible.

What we wanted as much as anything from the profession of medicine was that Heather be seen as a particular person, and a beautiful one at that, deserving all the best that science had to offer, but delivered with deep care and concentration. Just as Hippocrates taught his students millennia ago, the true art of medicine should be focused on the well-being of individual patients. It did much good for us. We were pleased that most of the caregivers we encountered saw Heather as the unique and special person she was. Dr. Emily Baiyee, her oncologist for the better part of two years, developed a relationship that seemed more like she was caring for a member of her family than a patient. Of course, Heather made that possible, given the way she carried herself throughout those years—as a shining example of her love of God and love for others.

Turning to the Bible

He who dwells in the shelter of the Most High, will abide in the shadow of the Almighty; I say to the Lord, "My refuge and my fortress, my God in whom I trust."

Psalm 91:1-2

Many friends reminded us of this psalm, and we turned to it often during our roller coaster journey. However, it would not have been helpful if we had gotten trapped in a flat interpretation of the psalm, and in so doing limited the multi-layered richness of its promises. If God says "no evil shall be allowed to befall you, no plague come near your tent" (v. 10), then a literal reading of that text was not applicable to our situation. How could we not "fear the terror of the night, nor the arrow that flies by day, nor the pestilence that stalks in the darkness, nor the destruction that wastes at the noonday" (v. 5-6) when already a fatal cancer had invaded Heather's body and entwined itself throughout her intestines? Would the hopes and promises of this psalm be available to us only if God miraculously healed Heather of this cancer, though every prognostic indicator said otherwise?

Of course, we never disbelieved in the power of God to do just that. But we refused to enclose God in such a tiny box. Rather, we were committed to believing the promises of this psalm were for us even if that did not happen. We had to believe that God would continue to be good to us within our circumstances. The psalmist writes: "Because he holds fast to me in love, I will deliver him; I will protect him, because he knows my name. When he calls to me, I will answer him; I will be with him in trouble; I will rescue him and honor him. With long life I will satisfy him and show him my salvation" (v. 14-16).

Wanting the full possibilities of these promises to be true, Heather and I depended on God to deliver us from this dark wood we were in. For us it was not a question of whether God could or would deliver, only how God would deliver. We hoped there would be other forms of deliverance in this life—even if the "long life" may not be in this life. In fact, it is far more likely it would be in the life to come. Even as we thought about the miraculous deliverance of Lazarus from the tomb—we remembered that his return from death to this life was only a temporary stay. However long a life he had afterward, Lazarus did one day die. What is more important in recalling the Lazarus story is the beautiful foreshadowing of what was to come, a resurrection unto eternal life.

To put it another way, most of us spend so much time thinking about the "little-l" *life* we have here that we begin to think this is all there is. How small our vision has become. What we truly want is the "big-L" *Life* that God offers us when we accept that Jesus is the resurrection and the life. In believing in him we will never die, and though one dies in this life, Life continues into eternity.

Remember: Martha *got it*. Heather *got it, too*. This is what Jesus was trying to say. I hope all of us will *get it*.

But for now, at the time of diagnosis, all we could think about was dwelling in the shelter of the Most High, abiding in the shadow of the almighty, and hiding under his wings for refuge. For to be honest, we were scared and just needed a safe place to rest.

For reflection and discussion

1. Are you the kind of person who wants to know the odds when you are trying to predict how something will turn out or would you rather take it as it comes?

2. What does it mean to know you are not a statistic but that you have your own particular path to forge?

3. How do you understand God's promises of deliverance? Do you expect complete healing or a full resolution of your problem as the only way God can answer your prayer?

4. When you face uncertainty, pain, and suffering, do you have trouble experiencing God as one who loves you as a unique and particular person and is always at work for good in your life?

4

Treatment Begins

*O Lord my God, I cried to you for help,
and you have healed me.*

Psalm 30:2

Less than a week after Heather's exploratory surgery, we met with an oncologist. Treatment options were explained and the usual first and best-researched three-drug chemotherapy regimen was recommended. The plan was to spread the chemotherapy out across twelve treatments, every two weeks for half a year.

As a physician, I felt obliged to look up the treatment options in an attempt to see if there were any other viable choices, or at the very least to assure myself we were on the right path. But deep down I knew that at this point in my life, I didn't want to be a physician searching for the right treatment, but a husband caring for his wife, relying on our doctors to make good decisions. By the grace of God, I was able to let go for the most part and trust. That was a true gift for someone like me who naturally wants to investigate every angle and think carefully and critically about everything.

On April 20, a Monday, Heather received her first course of chemotherapy at the out-patient oncology unit at Porter

Hospital in Denver. When that treatment concluded, the nurses connected her to an additional bag of chemotherapy and a shoulder harness so that it could slowly drip into her bloodstream over the next forty-eight hours at home.

Unfortunately, only six days after starting treatment, Heather's abdominal pain became critical. I faced my worst fear—that this cancer would advance to a fatal end before the chemotherapy could have any effect. Unable to eat and looking quite ill, Heather needed to go to the emergency room. It was a Saturday afternoon, and I was in for a big surprise. COVID restrictions were kicking in nationwide, and we were startled to find a new "no visitors" policy, prohibiting anyone from entering except the patient.

I felt sad and scared for Heather as I had to leave her at the emergency room that day. I had promised I would be with her through all that happened and already we were separated. Later that evening she was admitted to the hospital and placed on a treatment protocol for a small bowel obstruction. I knew this might be the case, but what I more deeply feared was that I might never see Heather alive again.

I panicked. I knew we belonged together at this time.

But here I was home alone, and there she was sick and alone in the hospital. As happened to many others, COVID was doing its devious work of disrupting people's lives and keeping people apart who belonged together.

I remember reaching out for prayer with several friends in my support network. My own prayers were far more desperate than anyone could know. I pleaded with God not to take Heather so soon!

I cried out with the psalmist:

> *My heart is in anguish within me;*
> *the terrors of death have fallen upon me.*
> *Fear and trembling come upon me,*
> *and horror overwhelms me.*

Psalm 55:4-5

I was simply not ready to let her go. I needed more time to care for her and be with her. Even if one day she would die from this cancer, I begged God to spare her life a little longer.

"Give us more time, Lord, please!"

The days ahead were hard, but God did hear our cries for mercy. First, the hospital relaxed its rules after a few days and one visitor was permitted. Seeing Heather again was a great relief—but my heart broke at her obvious discomfort. Unable to eat, she was receiving a full package of liquid nutrients through a central vein. Every day the surgeon saw her, waiting to see if the stranglehold of bowel obstruction would ease. The oncologist thought the best course of action was to operate. But to do so introduced a whole series of possible complications that could be lethal. Yet if the obstruction did not release itself, how would Heather survive?

As we wrestled with seemingly impossible choices, what I most remember was the patience of the surgeon. He knew better than anyone how complicated the surgery would be, trying to release numerous bowel loops from the masses of cancerous tumor that were scattered throughout her abdomen. Each time he visited with us, we asked what we should do—and each time he counseled caution.

One day, there were some small changes that suggested the obstruction might be lessening. Further improvements over the days that followed confirmed it. How grateful we were! It is hard to know exactly how this happened. She had only received one course of chemotherapy. Did that small amount start to work and shrink the tumor? Or did some other phenomena change the reality of the obstruction?

Ultimately, it did not matter *how*—only that Heather was experiencing some relief. To us, God had dramatically intervened in our lives. This was a miracle—and we knew that God deserved the praise.

Heather soon came home, still receiving her nutrition by vein, but at least with less pain, more strength, and the early return of an ability to swallow some liquids. She was back on chemotherapy, but additional complications over the next month included a blood clot to the lung that required a brief hospitalization and a massive lower leg swelling that improved over several weeks with some well-chosen medicines. Over and over, we felt blessed by the benefits of modern medicine, but even more had a deep gratitude to God for hearing our prayers and bringing her through these tumultuous times.

As Heather wrote to some friends when she left the hospital after the blood clot:

> I wish I could say I felt happy and hopeful that all will be well. My cousin used to say, "Life is not a straight line!" *But* I am confident that the Lord knows what lies ahead. Straight or crooked—He is not surprised, and He walks beside me. I even

had a dream the other night which reassured me of that.

… A couple of friends have reminded me of the story from Exodus 17 where the Israelite people were being attacked. Moses was on top of the hill praying with his arms stretched out to God. Whenever he held them up, the Israelites were winning, but when he got tired, they would fall down. Eventually, Aaron and Hur, his helpers, gave him a rock to sit on and each held up one of his arms until the battle was won that day.

The battle seems long—thank you for all the prayers and love and support on our behalf which hold us up!

When Heather and I looked back on this early experience of cancer treatment, we saw it as a Lazarus event. God had brought Heather back from the brink of death and given us a real hope for more time together. There was no promise of cure, nor any promise of how long things would continue to improve. Nevertheless, we knew God had heard our pleas. He had given back her life and given her back to me, at least for a time.

Challenges to biblical faith

As a privileged country in a Western society, we have learned to believe many things that are just not true. One of them is that everything is cause and effect: If you do X then you can be assured of Y. This assumption massively influences our view of modern medicine. If we take a treatment, like an antibiotic for pneumonia, for example, we "know" that we will get better from the pneumonia. And when we do, we are reinforced in our expectations that antibiotics cure pneumonia. But not everyone gets better after taking antibiotics for pneumonia.

The other view that holds significant ground for many is that life is simply random. What happens occurs by chance, and life is crazy and unpredictable. It doesn't matter what you do. Your only hope in a fickle universe is that sometimes things work out okay for us.

Between these two extremes lies a third way: In the beauty of God's natural created order, there is an ocean of associations that connect certain actions to reasonably predictable outcomes. Given the gift of our curiosity and intellect, humanity has discovered many of these secrets about how the world turns. Science has flourished in this milieu and discovered many of these associations. In the health arena, there are numerous examples that give wisdom and guidance for our health care choices. For example, while everyone who smokes does not get lung cancer, and some people who have never smoked get lung cancer, the large association between lung cancer and smoking should direct people to never start smoking or try to stop if they do.

Our choices matter. But the hard truth is they never matter as much as we may expect.

The chemotherapy, even though it was only one treatment, might have had some effect on the cancer that helped Heather get past this initial threat to her life. But our faith told us that it had to be more than simple cause and effect. And we certainly had no intention of considering it a random act of the universe. The outcome was a gift. For us, from our understanding of the biblical witness, God cared immensely about Heather's health and well-being, and God hears us when we cry out for help. It does not mean we always get what we ask. But when something good occurs, especially a sense of life being taken back from death, then as the people who saw Jesus' healing miracles, we should marvel at the power and love of God. The loss of the capacity for awe and wonder may be one of the more withering states of our modern soul.

Rather than taking anything for granted, we wanted to increase that capacity in ourselves in every way possible. Whatever was going to happen from here on, we were intent on looking for the goodness of God at work in this sickness. One day it might be a sickness unto death, that is, the death of the "little-l" life. But for now, it was sickness in life, and we would seek to nurture that life to the best of our ability, using whatever good might come from medicine, tightly bound to our faith in a good God.

Turning to the Bible

I will extol you, O Lord, for you have drawn me up
and have not let my foes rejoice over me.
O Lord my God, I cried to you for help,
and you have healed me.
O Lord, you have brought up my soul from the grave;
you restored me to life from among those who go down to the pit.
Sing praises to the Lord, O you his saints,
and give thanks to his holy name.

Psalm 30:1-4

When Heather came home from the hospital, this was the psalm that best explained what happened for us. We had arrived at death's door and were in danger of falling into the pit of no return. But like the psalmist, God's healing hand brought Heather back from the grave.

How good that she came back home! How wonderful that the familiarity of our family surroundings could ease her troubles and add to her comforts!

This psalm, like many others, encourages us to call out to God in our troubles—because God hears us when we call. As one friend said when dealing with a new diagnosis of cancer, "I just need to know that he sees me and hears me."

When Hagar fled from Sarai's mistreatment in Genesis 16, an angel of the Lord found Hagar near a spring in the desert and spoke words of assurance that God had not forgotten her. Hagar named that well Beer Lahai Roi, the well of "the Living One who sees me."

When Moses met God at the burning bush, the Lord said to him "I have surely seen the affliction of my people who are in Egypt and have heard their cry because of their taskmasters. I know their sufferings and I have come down to deliver them" (Exodus 3:7-8).

We may not know what God's deliverance will look like. We may not even know if it will come in this life. Yet when we feel like "the cords of death encompassed me; the torrents of destruction assailed me" (Psalm 18:4), it makes all the difference to trust in the reassurance of a passage like Psalm 30.

These psalms make bold assertions that the God who hears and sees is also the God who acts. The same God who met Hagar in the desert and rescued the Israelites from the hands of the Egyptians is listening to us. Indeed, it can be troubling to observe sometimes how slowly God acts. In our first brush with Heather's mortality, we were blessed with what we recognized as God's immediate and dramatic response to our prayers. We knew from others' experiences that it doesn't always happen that way. It would not always be that way for us. There were times to come when a seemingly silent God would greatly test our faith.

For reflection and discussion

1. How do you and your family think about the relationship between God's compassionate care for us and the wisdom of medical science?
2. When you pray for loved ones undergoing medical treatment, what kinds of things do you say to God? And what has been your experience in these crises?
3. Have you ever reached a point of real terror and desperate "crying out" to God?
4. What Scriptures have helped you in these crises?

5

A Good Response to Treatment

Hope is the power of being cheerful in circumstances we know to be desperate.

G. K. Chesterton

After escaping numerous pitfalls in the first two months of treatment, we settled into a routine common to many patients with cancer. Everything revolved around the dates of treatment—planned for months in advance. In Heather's case, every two weeks we knew where she would be, barring any complications—in the chair in the treatment center, hooked up to the tubes that slowly and carefully dripped the medicine into her body over three to five hours.

Heather naturally grew tired of going. Each time we went, she gathered her strength and directed her focus on accepting this as her task. It was good we did not know how much and for how long our lives would be ruled by this schedule. But we knew it was going to be for a long time if it was successful.

People asked, "When will you be finished with treatment?"

They had a hard time understanding that there was no end to Heather's course of treatment. In our case, we would only stop treatment when it was no longer working. If we let up, in Heather's case, we knew that this cancer would grow back with surprising force and speed.

I was continually amazed, given how hard I knew it was for Heather to gather her strength for each visit, that she interacted with our caregivers in such a caring way. Since she was a nurse herself, she felt most connected with her nurses. Despite her circumstances, she sought to be her usual self, asking them about their lives and how their families were doing. Because of her natural concern for them, our caregivers came to know Heather and deeply care for her in a special way.

At the end of six months, Heather had finished a full course of this initial three-drug cocktail. Given the cumulative toxicity of platinum-based chemotherapy, it was known that beyond these twelve treatments the risk of allergic reactions would become quite high if Heather was exposed to further platinum. At this point in the journey, other than the seventy-two-hour period from Monday to Wednesday every two weeks, Heather had reasonably good energy for visiting family and friends, enjoying holidays, taking bike rides and hikes, and eating with appreciation for the goodness of food. The scans by the end of treatment were very encouraging, the tumor having been reduced to only one small area at the original site of the cancer in the upper portion of her stomach.

Heather wrote in her CaringBridge journal during this time:

> We truly credit God's graciousness in using and guiding the chemo to good effect and thank and praise Him for the measure of healing that I'm

> experiencing now. We know God has heard the prayers of many—and has in His love, given this gift ...
>
> Bob and I see God at work in wonderful ways. ...
>
> For right now, without sticking our heads in the sand—we know what gastric cancer can lead to—we are choosing to live in the present—to be grateful for the measure of health God has given me and we will leave the future in His hands, knowing He is already there and will give us grace and strength for life and health as the future unfolds.

Given the good response, our oncologist recommended a daily dose of an oral drug in an effort to maintain control without the risks of a more intense secondary regimen. This went on for about three months of apparent stability, lulling us into a routine that almost made us forget Heather had cancer.

Of course, we never did forget. We continued playing a cat and mouse game with COVID that was a constant reminder. Each time we thought about doing something outside the house, it was only after surveying the terrain with senses on high alert for any dangerous encounter with someone with the virus. If we planned a visit with the grandchildren, that hope could be dashed if we heard someone in the family had a fever or a cough or some symptom that could be passed on to Heather. Many times, we bundled up with family members and friends and met outdoors and at a distance. Better to have met in whatever way we could than never to have met at all, we always said.

This hypervigilance was wearing. I took it as my responsibility to protect Heather, so I became the most watchful one. Often, I wondered if I struck the right balance. Too much protection and she never would see anyone. Not enough protection and I don't know if I could have forgiven myself if she had gotten sick. By God's grace, she never did get COVID. In these cases, how much depends on our choices is never fully known. We simply tried to act reasonably, asked others to likewise be thoughtful about Heather's susceptibility, and ultimately trusted God to watch over us with his goodness and love.

Think back to Psalm 91 in Chapter 3 for a moment. Verse 3 even says that God will protect us from "deadly pestilence." If we had understood that passage literally, then why would we even worry about COVID? Or any other infectious disease, for that matter?

But we understood that such a simplistic view of Scripture was exactly what Satan was using when he tempted Jesus in the wilderness, a story so important that it shows up in three of the four Gospels (Matthew 4 and Luke 4 with a brief recap in Mark 1). In the longer versions, Satan and Jesus are atop the pinnacle of the temple. Here Satan tries to tempt Jesus to test God's protective power using the very words of Psalm 91. Satan taunts Jesus: "If you are the Son of God, throw yourself down from here, for it is written, 'He will command his angels concerning you, to guard you,' and 'On their hands they will bear you up, lest you strike your foot against a stone.'"

But Jesus, of course, saw through this misuse of God's promise and protection. One does not act foolishly and take unnecessary risks. That idea of testing God is strongly spoken against in Scripture.

For us, the promises of Psalm 91 did not mean Heather would never get COVID. We believed God gave us reason and thought to discern a balance of risk and benefit, avoiding unnecessary exposure to COVID while still finding time to be with others. We never thought God promised that dangers other than cancer would never beset us. We were still in the world of evil and harmful things.

Challenges to biblical faith

"Why did this happen to me?"

That's a challenging question we all face at some point in our lives. We heard some version of this question from friends many times: Why did Heather, in very good health, doing good work as the school nurse at a charter school for pregnant and parenting teens, suddenly get a life-threatening cancer?

In our case, some would even go so far as to say she didn't deserve it, especially for one who had been so faithful throughout her life loving God and serving the poor and needy of this world.

"Why would God let this happen to her?"

I must be clear that this was never Heather's thought. As you may remember from her journaling, quoted earlier, she did not waste time with "why?" but rather asked "what for?" Heather was always pointing people toward the greater question: "What might God do in and through me because of this illness?"

In fact, one of her heroes was a friend we knew when we worked at a mission to the homeless in Washington, D.C. over twenty-five years earlier. She was diagnosed with ovarian cancer in her early sixties and later died from that cancer. When she was asked, she always responded to the question of "why you?" with the disarming counter "why not me?"

And isn't that the more appropriate response! Look at the world, where tragedy and trouble are always apparent somewhere. Look at the paths of people throughout the Bible. Look at the history of the chosen people, Israel—from the wanderings of patriarchs to slavery in Egypt, forty years in the desert and later exile, living as strangers in a foreign land.

Troubles, pain, and affliction are the mark of being human, from biblical history to the present day. But somehow, we delude ourselves into thinking otherwise. We do all we can to buffer ourselves from the world around us, creating a much smaller world of our own making where we think we have control, believing what happens to others outside our buffer zone won't happen to us.

Perhaps we have been lulled into thinking we have such power over sickness and disease that whatever happens, it can be fixed. Or perhaps we overlay such naïve invulnerability with a light coating of religion and assume God would never allow such things to happen to us.

But here we come to the heart of the matter. God could have chosen to manipulate the universe so that no one would ever suffer—but that is not what God did. At a much higher price, God chose to enter into our world and suffer with it. God chose not to protect us from all harm, but to be with us in whatever harm befalls us.

Undergirded by our biblical faith, we can face our vulnerability to sickness, suffering, and death as creatures in a fallen world. Jesus told us to expect troubles, and at the same time be strengthened in knowing it would not happen apart from his victory over death. "In the world you will have tribulation," Jesus tells us in John 16:33, "But take heart; I have overcome the world."

So how do we strengthen our faith to live in a world of troubles and trials? Heather and I found that one pillar was joining with friends in prayer.

Turning to the Bible

Consider Philippians 1:3-7:

> I thank my God in all my remembrance of you, always in every prayer of mine for you all making my prayer with joy, because of your partnership in the gospel from the first day until now. And I am sure of this, that he who began a good work in you will bring it to completion at the day of Jesus Christ. It is right for me to feel this way because I hold you in my heart, for you are all partakers with me of grace.

When close friends of ours first suggested inviting us to a prayer meeting (remotely, given the COVID risk), we were at first unsure how to respond. They wanted to gather friends near and far to plead for mercy and grace for Heather and me during our difficult journey. At first, we wondered if we had the energy for this, but we decided to accept the invitation.

How fortunate it was that we let go—and let God! We had a series of prayer meetings over these first six months, and others later on when the need arose. Every time was a blessing. These friends who joined us in prayer, like Paul, held us in their hearts. The tenderness and warmth of being held like that did much to buoy our spirits. Before that, with the isolation of COVID and the minimal interaction we had with others given how sick Heather was, we felt very alone.

Seeing our friends, even remotely, and experiencing their deep concern for us, eased the weight we were carrying. At the time, Heather added this note to her CaringBridge journal:

> I see God at work—through the prayers and expressions of love and support from Bob, my family, and so many friends, through the work of medicine and good medical care, and I pray that I will be patient and hopeful as I continue letting the treatment work in me. I am overwhelmed and humbled by the love and prayers and support from so many people all over the world standing with Bob and me in this time.
>
> To me, it feels like a glimpse of what Heaven will be like!

Reflecting back on our hesitancy to join the online prayer meetings, I think we were afraid of how difficult it would be to be transparent and vulnerable and share our pain with others. But that turned out to be a false fear once we were in their presence. Their tears, their honest crying out to God on our behalf, and their frank request that Jesus be in our midst as he had promised he would be (Matthew 18:20), made being vulnerable both natural and good.

"It's a glimpse of heaven," Heather said.

Tears quickly became a regular part of our lives. We found out how particularly good it is crying with those who love you. This was all very new for me, having cried so rarely before in my life. Little did I realize how easily and without warning tears would come to a stoic like me until I entered this new world of grief and sadness and shared it with others. It changed the way I looked at things.

Philosopher and theologian Nicholas Wolterstorff described his own changing understanding of tears after the death of his son: "I shall look at the world through tears. Perhaps I will see things that dry-eyed I could not see."

When Heather and I were married on February 14, 1986, we had engraved on our wedding bands: "Phil 1:6." From the above-quoted passage, it says, "And I am sure of this, that he who began a good work in you will bring it to completion on the day of Christ Jesus." That day we saw our lives beginning together no longer as two but one, and believed God who began it would also complete it. Having this trust in God to finish the work of our marriage remained with us throughout the ordeal that one day would take Heather home to be with him. What I did not know was how much I was going to struggle when the time came to let her go.

For reflection and discussion

1. What does it mean to have someone hold you in their heart, the way Paul held the people in the Philippian church in his heart?
2. What questions have you heard friends and family raise when someone you love becomes seriously ill? What questions have you asked? In light of this chapter, and these readings from Scripture, are you rethinking any of those questions?
3. Do you find yourself worrying about your own future health? How do you cope with such worries?
4. In your life, do you know someone who will listen to your fears and questions and respond in a supportive way?
5. Have you experienced being in the center of a circle of prayer during a crisis you've faced? What happened?

Another Encounter With Death

The capacity to wonder is among man's greatest gifts.
Christian philosopher Josef Pieper

As Thanksgiving rolled around and we moved toward the end of 2020, things seemed to be going fairly well. Heather was quite upbeat in her post to friends and family:

> Happy Thanksgiving to you! What a year for all of us!
>
> I know this Thanksgiving looks different for almost all of us this year and that so many things/travel/events/celebrations have been put on hold or have looked very different in 2020. Still, this is a time for us to reflect on what we are thankful for and for God's blessings to us in the past year.
>
> I have so much to be grateful for this year! Seven months ago, I was in pretty bad shape. Learning of the cancer diagnosis, we wondered if the chemo was going to help. It did—remarkably! As you've seen from my posts, I've felt pretty well

and have had great times with our family and friends, even with social distancing. A real lifeline and encouragement has been connecting with so many friends over these past few months and the incredible blessing of prayers and words of support and fellowship.

On Heather's birthday, December 27—surprised that it was even a possibility given where we had been a few months before—we went cross-country skiing, a tradition we had over many years. But afterward Heather did not feel well and each day felt more pain, more weakness, and more inability to eat. The doctor quickly arranged another CT scan and on New Year's Eve we learned the cancer was spreading throughout her small bowel once again.

Despite that sad news, Heather was still able to have hope as she posted to our friends and family on December 31:

> So, on this eve of the new year, I'm thankful. Firstly—we made it through this strange and difficult year—I believe there were even some blessings in the midst of the restrictions. I'm thankful for good and swift medical care. I'm thankful for the measure of time and good health God has blessed me with. I'm thankful for family and friends both near and far away—YOU!—for caring and loving and praying for Bob and me! We appreciate that more than you can imagine!! I'm thankful for Bob—my constant companion, caregiver, supporter, advocate, and love of my life, who is walking with me through every bit of this. And Bob and I are sustained by the Lord who

knows our suffering, holds us close when we feel afraid and gives us hope in His promise of Life.

Despite Heather's unflagging spirit, the next few weeks were very difficult. Heather was quickly getting sick again. On January 4, because of the aggressive return of the cancer, the oncologist decided to return to the platinum-based therapy despite its risks. It was a time when we looked to Scripture, specifically Psalm 33:18-19:

> *Behold, the eye of the Lord is on those who fear him,*
> *on those whose hope is in his steadfast love,*
> *that he may deliver their soul from death.*

Unfortunately, but not unpredictably, she was only able to tolerate this regimen for a few short weeks. One Monday morning, the dreaded and severe allergic reaction suddenly occurred, requiring immediate action on the nurses' part to reverse it. That was a scary moment—but it passed quickly.

We were left with the more frightening questions: Was there another option that had the potential to hinder the cancer's spread? Would it be tolerable? Would there be time to see it work? Seeing Heather looking as if the cords of death were entangling her once again, I became frightened.

As in earlier crises, Psalms made so much sense to me. I cried from the depths of my soul for God to come and save us. Underneath our anguish, we knew our greatest hope was in God, and once again found Psalms putting our deepest feelings into words:

> *Whom have I in heaven but you?*
> *And there is nothing on earth that I desire besides you.*

> *My flesh and my heart may fail,*
> *but God is the strength of my heart and my portion forever.*
>
> **Psalm 73:25-26**

Whatever the physical realities, we wanted with all our hearts to believe we had a refuge and defender from heaven.

What happened over the next two months was a wonderful surprise! It was difficult to see until the new treatment—an immunotherapy—had a chance to take effect, but eventually we realized that Heather was being given another experience of the miraculous. We thought of it as seeing Lazarus released from the grave for a second time! This was something we could not have expected simply based on data. As a new treatment for gastric cancer, there was only limited evidence to support its benefit. But, in the goodness of God, it took Heather back from death's door and returned her to the land of the living. In fact, she began to tolerate this phase of treatment even better than the first one. The cancer once again regressed. Heather could eat again, regain her energy, and suffer little or no pain.

Thinking of where we were only three months before at the turn of the new year, it felt appropriate to join the psalmist in song:

> *But I will sing of your strength;*
> *I will sing aloud of your steadfast love in the morning.*
> *For you have been to me a fortress*
> *and a refuge in the day of my distress.*
> *O my Strength, I will sing praises to you,*
> *for you, O God, are my fortress,*
> *the God who shows me steadfast love.*
>
> **Psalm 59: 16-17**

That this happened at all was remarkable enough. That it continued for the remainder of the year was an extraordinary gift of God. Heather's body and spirit, despite the existence of cancer for over one year now, was showing great resilience and strength.

At one point, she posted:

> "God is able to do immeasurably more than all we ask or imagine, according to his power that is at work within us! To him be glory!"
>
> **Ephesians 3:20**
>
> This is the reality that Bob and I are experiencing this summer. My lab tests and recent CT scan all show a diminishing of the cancer's activity and I have good energy and am feeling well! This response is way beyond what's normally expected with stage 4 stomach cancer. We are so grateful! We've been enjoying summer weather, eating dinner in our backyard, and spending time with our kids and grandkids—including three birthdays!

Then a little later in the year, she wrote:

> It's hard to believe that it has been eighteen months since I was diagnosed with stomach cancer. I'm so happy to report that my CT scan last week showed no cancer outside my stomach! The combination of the chemo and immunotherapy drugs has really been working for me by reducing the amount of cancer and holding it at bay. By

all accounts, I'm "an outlier"—in a positive sense! Bob and I don't take this for granted and continue to be thankful to God's graciousness to us for the health and well-being given. I'm thankful for excellent medical care and that it's effective, and I'm thankful for competent, caring doctors and nurses.

As this roller coaster year of 2021 closed, she wrote on New Year's Eve:

> Even the doctors are telling us we are in uncharted territory as so few people with my stage of stomach cancer have done this well. We are thankful for how God has led us and been with us over the years. He has been with us in some very hard things and brought many blessings, like now—above and beyond what is expected! We don't know what the new year holds but we are confident that God walks with us and also are so thankful for all of you who bless and encourage us in so many ways!!

The new year of 2022, like 2021, was going to be another "grab each other and hold tight" ride on the roller coaster. But we knew how much we had come through, and Psalms kept giving us the words to say that would steady our hearts for what lay ahead:

> *For you have delivered my soul from death,*
> *yes, my feet from falling,*
> *that I may walk before God in the light of life.*
>
> **Psalm 56:13**

Challenges to biblical faith

A great cultural challenge in our age of medical success is to see health as a possession—an entitlement we own and control—rather than as a gift.

As songwriter Neil Young put it:

> Love is a rose but you better not pick it
> Only grows when it's on the vine
> Handful of thorns and you'll know you've missed it
> Lose your love when you say the word mine

German Catholic philosopher Josef Pieper described the challenge for Christians in his book, *Leisure, The Basis of Culture*:

> We have only to think for a moment how much the Christian understanding of life depends upon the existence of "Grace"; let us recall that the Holy Spirit of God is himself called a 'gift' in a special sense; that the great teachers of Christianity say that the premise of God's justice is his love; that everything gained and everything claimed follows upon something given, and comes after something gratuitous and unearned; that in the beginning there is always a gift.

When we act as if our health is something we can control as a possession, then our attitude becomes expectant and demanding. We assume we will get better. We demand medicine do its job and cure us when we are sick. When things do not go well, we angrily conclude someone is at fault and look for who to blame.

In contrast there is the choice to be grateful for what is given. Each time Heather got sick to the point of death, we had hope that something could change that trajectory. Yet we never had control over whether it did. We prayed, and fervently, along with many others who cared for us on this journey. Trusting God was our firmest foundation. And when her body took a healthy turn, we could only be thankful for God's kindness and grace.

If I might briefly put back on my doctor's hat, there is good evidence that having an attitude of gratitude and marvel is one of the healthiest things we can do. Instead of demanding with gritted teeth and tight fists, we remain open to surprise, delighted by wonder, and attentive to the gracious ways of God in a broken world.

As biblical theologian Walter Brueggemann describes the connection in his book *Living Toward a Vision*:

> Our penchant for control and predictability, our commitment to quantity, our pursuit of stability and security—all this gives us a sense of priority and an agenda that is concerned to reduce the element of surprise and newness in our lives. And when newness and surprise fail, there is not likely to be graciousness, healing, or joy. Enough critics have made the point that when experiences of surprise and newness are silenced in our lives, there is no amazement, and where there is no amazement, there cannot be the full coming to health, wholeness, and maturity.

It was obvious already at this stage in our journey that there was no option for control, predictability, or stability. So why not leave room for surprise and amazement? God had already amazed us twice in pulling Heather back from death to life.

Thus, we knew that our goal throughout this long journey with cancer was to remain open to what God might do. And what we discovered was how needful it would be to surround ourselves daily with the promises of Scripture if we were to "give thanks in all circumstances, for this is the will of God in Christ Jesus for you" (I Thessalonians 5:18).

Turning to the Bible

I love the Lord, because he has heard
my voice and my pleas for mercy.
Because he inclined his ear to me,
therefore I will call upon him as long as I live.
The snares of death encompassed me;
The pangs of the grave laid hold of me;
I suffered distress and anguish.
Then I called on the name of the Lord:
"Lord, I pray, deliver my soul!"

Psalm 116:1-4

On at least four different levels, the first half of Psalm 116 spoke directly to our most recent circumstances. In fact, I commend all nineteen verses to you—and we will return to consider the second half of Psalm 116 later in this book.

First, we recognized that the psalmist was in the same frightful situation as we were, overcome by his closeness with death.

Second, he cries out to God in language that clearly reflects his belief that God is his only hope. In our day and age, we have many places where we might put our hope: in the doctors, in the medicines, or in a belief that an incurable cancer might soon be curable with new research unearthing new treatments. But regardless of the varying value of each of these pieces, when most desperate, like the psalmist, we knew our surest hope was in God.

Third, the psalmist does not take his deliverance for granted. He is astounded by the marvel of the full and free salvation that has been granted by God. We too sought the same posture.

Finally, as a result of this deliverance from great peril, the psalmist comes to a firm conclusion: "Because he has turned his ear to me, I will call on him as long as I live" (v. 2). Our growing belief was that turning to God for help must be our main response if we would have any chance of keeping our footing in the shifting sands that lay ahead.

For reflection and discussion

1. Do you tend to take your health for granted? Are you surprised when sickness arises or your body fails?
2. What has caused you to experience wonderment in your life? How can you nurture a sense of amazement and marvel at the ways you might experience God in your life?

3. What role does gratitude play in your life? Are there ways you practice gratitude—or teach gratitude to others like your children?

4. Do you have a favorite psalm to which you turn in times of crisis? Or is there another passage from the Bible you recall in hard times?

7

The End of Treatment

The greater our medical successes, the more unacceptable is failure, and the more intolerable and frightening is death.

Bioethicist Leon Kass

Early 2022 went well. Months went by with good health most days of the week except a slowdown for two days every two weeks when Heather was receiving treatment. By the middle of the year, Heather posted this encouraging news:

> The wonderful thing is that while Bob and I live within certain limitations these days, thankfully the treatment I'm receiving every other week is holding the cancer stable … This is reason to rejoice—and even the medical team is amazed at how my body is responding to the treatment! Cancer is hard—I have some friends and family members also going through treatment and, for each person, the uncertainty is one of the hardest parts—is the treatment helping? What will the scan say? How will my body feel today? Not taking any of it for granted, Bob and I thank God for His graciousness in allowing me to enjoy such

good health in these days and we appreciate so much the good medical care—and the support and prayers of so many!

What was especially good during this period of prolonged benefit was the energy Heather had to be with family and friends. It was gratifying to see her with the four grandchildren, all who were less than four years old when Heather was diagnosed in 2020. Now they had time to grow and to get to know their "Nina" a bit more. Before that, their memory would have been very small indeed. We saw that God was kind, and he was permitting the time that would one day allow these four little people to remember their grandmother better.

Yet this was stability, not cure, and as expected, this gracious time of health had an endpoint coming. However, all during this time, though I was not consciously aware of it, my brain was always on some level of high alert. I mostly internalized it, putting a stress on my mind and body that was not healthy. In some ways, as I marveled at Heather's energy on good days and watched with gratitude for how she invested herself in caring for others, I had no choice but to keep this tension within. Deep down I was already grieving—even though the event of Heather's death that would most sadden me had not even happened.

Sometime in August, we received news that the tumor markers were up, reflecting that the cancer was spreading again. We had already been through this twice before. For a third time something new had to be tried, but the options had shrunk and looked far less optimistic.

Heather summarized well where we found ourselves with the new results:

> Unfortunately, this time, the scan showed some spots in my abdomen and lungs where the cancer has spread. Needless to say, while we knew this might happen one day, it still felt like a punch to the gut! It means the treatment I've been on for the past year and a half, which was fairly easy to deal with, is no longer working. We are so thankful to have had that wonderful space of good health.
>
> On Monday, I will begin a new treatment regimen ... There are a lot of unknowns; particularly in how well the cancer will respond to the treatment and how my body will react to the potential toxic side effects of the two new medicines.
>
> We are hopeful that since my body is quite strong right now and I've tolerated previous ones well, that things will go OK. BUT we would truly appreciate your prayers for us as I go into what we're calling "Phase 3" of my cancer treatment. I may be the one going through the chemo but Bob, as the one walking with me every day, feels the burden of all of this very deeply. We know we can't do this in our own strength, but we also know that God is FOR us, that God already knows the outcome and is with us. What we are praying for most of all is that God would give us a deep sense of peace—God's peace. The kind that goes beyond feelings of the moment and potential outcomes and is that peace beyond human understanding.

> We sense a measure of that now but know we will need it in increasing measure in the days ahead.

"Phase 3" worked, but just a little and only for a short time. The ups and downs of the roller coaster were starting to wear us out, as Heather posted:

> September was a hard month for us. I was tolerating the new phase 3 chemo regimen pretty well but the lab markers that track the cancer growth were equivocal, so we weren't sure if the chemo was working. Besides that, this was really the last in the line of available chemo and after that … well, let's just say we know we're running out of options … Bob and I were both kind of stressed. Our bodies were feeling it physically and we maybe were a little short with each other at times. But WOW, we had to straighten out our "stinkin' thinkin'"!!! God has been so faithful all along the way! He has helped us through much more difficult situations. He has numbered our days and He will carry us through all of them!

For me, it felt like we were moving toward the end of a long journey, and honestly, like the psalmist, I was physically and spiritually drained:

> *Be gracious to me, O God, for I am in distress;*
> *my eye is wasted from grief;*
> *my soul and my body also.*
> *For my life is spent in sorrow,*
> *and my years with sighing;*

> *my strength fails because of my iniquity,*
> *and my bones waste away.*
>
> **Psalm 31: 9-10**

It seemed for so long we had been struggling, and now things were about to move toward an end we knew one day would come.

But it doesn't matter what you think you know before that day arrives. You can never truly be ready when it comes.

As a last look at any possibility for treatment benefit, we were referred and transferred our care to the academic medical center at the University of Colorado. Our new oncologist, Dr. Sunnie Kim, quickly became a source of wisdom and true care as the weeks advanced with primarily bad news that the cancer was growing. Heather's obstruction worsened, though was still only partial. Her body was weakening quickly.

We went through all the protocols necessary for entering an experimental trial. Planned to begin in December, the schedule was mapped out and placed in the calendar for the next several weeks. Heather posted again on her CaringBridge site:

> I am receiving very caring and competent treatment which we appreciate very much. Still, our hope is in God, who knows every detail of my cancer and is going before us, guiding and directing our path and walking with us in it. We believe this study is the next right step to take and will see how it goes.
>
> It's just a week until Thanksgiving! We truly are thankful for so many blessings despite cancer in

these past few years, including reconnecting with so many of you!

On November 30, we met with Dr. Kim. It was the meeting we had been dreading. At least we were blessed with a doctor who could be honest, candid, and caring. It was time to stop treatment, she said. Heather's body was too weak and the side effects of the experimental treatment would be too strong, robbing her of any quality of life while her quantity of life was shrinking rapidly. Though it was not what we wanted to hear, we understood what she was saying.

Stepping aside for a moment from the intensity and emotion in the doctor's office, in a negative sense, one can look on these times as an act of giving up. But that is never the way we saw it. Dealing with cancer these last three years, at times it felt like it was the main force controlling our lives. But as we turned from treatment to no treatment, we knew deep down that the cancer was never in control. God had continued to work out his purposes for Heather's life. We had often sustained ourselves during the unexpected twists and turns and all the uncertainties of cancer care by a sense that Heather's days were numbered, not by the cancer, but by God.

As a cautionary note, this does not mean we believed God sent this horrible cancer into Heather's life. Cancer is an evil and destructive reality that inflicts much harm upon many people. All sickness is a deviation from God's original plan, and throughout Jesus' earthly ministry he sought to heal those who suffered from numerous bodily and mental ailments. This reveals both God's opposition to and authority over every form of sickness. Despite the hostile forces of disease, we should not be tempted to think they are what control our lives. Though Heather's cancer was a powerful and harsh reality, we refused to believe it had dominion over her life. God's plan for Heather was never thwarted. Rather, God entered into this experience of cancer with us and fulfilled his purposes for us not despite it but in the midst of it. In all the troubling circumstances of our lives, God is about redeeming what evil seeks to destroy.

How often we returned to Psalm 139 to remind us of this truth:

> *I praise you, for I am fearfully and wonderfully made ...*
> *My frame was not hidden from you*
> *when I was being made in secret,*
> *intricately woven in the depths of the earth.*
> *Your eyes saw my unformed substance;*
> *in your book were written every one of them,*
> *the days that were formed for me,*
> *when as yet there was none of them.*
>
> **Psalm 139:14-16**

Back in the doctor's room, we accepted what was said. We cried in the face of its truth and reality. And we prepared for our last phase—to do all that was possible to help Heather feel less pain and more comfort for the days that remained.

Challenges to biblical faith

How do you know when the time has come to let go of this life and face death? How do you find a way to cherish this life but refuse to cling to it as if this is all there is? How do you find the way in-between, neither holding onto life too tightly nor letting it go too easily? In our current age, with so much power and control over life compared to previous generations, it is easy to lose our balance.

Of course, it has never been easy to face our mortality or talk about death.

"Neither the sun nor death can be stared at directly," French moralist François de La Rochefoucauld wrote in the seventeenth century—and it is just as true today.

But in our day, we have developed the uncanny ability to not look at all. What distinguishes us from our ancestors is the power of technology to overcome sickness and death. It is a wonderful age that we live in, one of unprecedented skill in diagnosing and treating disease. Perhaps we do not realize how recent the phenomenon is, with most of our progress achieved only within the last hundred years. The physician and prolific author Lewis Thomas, writing about his training at Boston City Hospital, reflected on how much they knew about disease in the 1930s but how little they could do.

> On the wards of the great Boston teaching hospitals … it gradually dawned on us that we didn't know much that was really useful, that we could do nothing to change the course of the great majority of the diseases we were so busily analyzing, that medicine, for all its façade as a learned profession, was in real life a profoundly ignorant occupation.

Indeed, it was still the basics of kindly care, just as it had always been, that made any difference. Thomas wrote:

> If being in a hospital bed made a difference, it was mostly the difference produced by warmth, shelter, and food, and attentive, friendly care, and all the matchless skill of the nurses in providing these things. Whether you survived or not depended on the natural history of the disease itself. Medicine made little or no difference.

Serving my internship in this same hospital almost fifty years later, I can assure you that our perspective had changed dramatically. Refusing any passive acceptance, we ran about frantically ordering tests and instituting treatments with the sole goal of defeating the enemy. And often we did, only increasing our resolve to push it further into oblivion.

It seems there is a connection between our capabilities to overcome disease and our difficulty in facing death. We learn to depend on our technical prowess to get us out of the next jam, whether because of how well things turned out before, or how well things went for someone else, or just because of how much medicine can offer and how much our culture believes in its power. But in winning so many battles, we fail to realize that someday we will need to let go. This puts medicine in danger of making promises it cannot keep and causes confusion about where true salvation lies. As I wrote in my earlier book, "Modern medicine as well as the community that supports it have become confused about its purpose and transferred hope for salvation from the halls of faith to the corridors of medicine."

"Do not go gentle into that good night," Dylan Thomas advised in a poem he penned as he watched the weakening of age in his previously strong and militant father. And surely there is a time for that kind of resistance. But neither is it always good, and the time will come when to "rage, rage against the dying of the light" will be counterproductive to living well at the end.

Dante, reflecting an image from Cicero's *On Old Age* centuries earlier, spoke of a traveler at the end of life who, like a good sailor approaching port, lowers his sail and moves gently into dock as the boat arrives at a site of repose after a long journey. To "rage" at this final stage was an untimely aggression that only ended in shipwreck. Dante wrote:

> O you miserable and debased beings who speed into this port with sails raised high! Where you should take your rest, you shipwreck yourselves against the force of the wind and perish at the very place to which you have been so long journeying.

We were lucky, Heather and I. We had received wonderful medical care over the last three years. Much of the treatment we received was highly beneficial. But we never thought medicine could save us. We had talked much about this day before the time came. And fortunately, we had a doctor courageous enough to tell us the truth when the time had come for its telling.

We had come to understand through many experiences watching others' lives as medical practitioners, as well as what happened in our own lives, that in its fullest form Heather's health, my health, the health of anyone and everyone, must encompass both life and death. And that only happens by way of love. As Wendell Berry expresses it:

> Any definition of health that is not silly must include death. The world of love includes death, suffers it, and triumphs over it. The world of efficiency is defeated by death; at death, all its instruments and procedures stop. The world of love continues, and of this grief is the proof.

There is no question that the love I and many others had for Heather had made a significant difference on the journey leading up to the day when we turned from treatment to comfort care. Now it was time, on approaching port, to lower the sails and move gently into dock, to a place of repose after a long journey. Truly our love would be stretched to the limit as we sought to guide Heather to shore.

Turning to the Bible

It is the Lord who goes before you.
He will be with you; he will not leave you or forsake you.
Do not fear or be dismayed.

Deuteronomy 31:8

Several times in Heather's posts during this time she spoke of the ability to move forward because:

"God already knows the outcome."

"He has gone before us and will guide us."

God "is going before us, guiding and directing our path and walking with us in it."

This idea of God's omnipresence, most directly understood as his ability to be present everywhere at the same time, is expressed beautifully in Psalm 139. No matter where the psalmist goes, whether to the heights of heaven, the depths of hell, or the uttermost parts of the sea, God is already there. But God being an eternal being, that omnipresence is not just in space—but in time. If we could run into the future, we would find God already there. This is a most reassuring part of the character of God, and for Heather and me this was a life-giving and empowering truth. We had watched people approach death and die in our roles as doctor and nurse. But that experience does not change the unknowingness of what we were about to experience. Knowing that God already was "up ahead" steadied our souls and anchored our hope.

In Exodus 3, God tells Moses at the burning bush that he is to go to Pharoah and ask for the release of His people. Moses then asks, "If I come to the people of Israel and say to them, 'The God of your fathers has sent me to you,' and they ask me, 'What is his name?' what shall I say to them?"

Then God said to Moses, "I AM WHO I AM." Others have suggested the translation from Hebrew could include, "I AM WHAT I AM," or "I WILL BE WHAT I WILL BE." I don't think it stretches too much to add "I WILL BE THERE WHEN YOU GET THERE." It is all about the character of God, one who defines himself by himself. Resisting any of our efforts to put God in a box of our own making, this allows for an understanding of God's power and God's love far beyond anything we could ask or imagine.

Again, as Psalm 139 also reminds us, even if I run into darkness, "the darkness is not dark to you; the night is as bright as the day, for darkness is as light with you" (Psalm 139:12).

Our immediate future seemed dark indeed—but it made a big difference to believe God was already there.

Nothing that happened to us could extinguish the love and light of God.

For reflection and discussion

1. Have you experienced a time when a family member or close friend was nearing the end of life? Was it difficult to know when to fight and when to let go?
2. Why do so many see letting go as giving up? What are some of the influences from our culture that you see contributing to that attitude?
3. How can you increase your sensitivity to God's timing in life and death? What Scriptures help you to understand these questions from God's perspective?
4. Do you find it hard to support family and friends when there is no way to "fix" their suffering?

8

Crossing Over

Life is a gift which death does not vitiate or void.
William Stringfellow

By December 2022, Heather was clear in her thinking: As her days wound down, she did not want to be in a hospital but home amongst familiarity, family, and friends. We did accept a brief hospitalization under doctor's advice that a small procedure might relieve some of Heather's intestinal blockage, but it did not turn out to be helpful. Shortly after returning home, we engaged the services of hospice.

As we entered into this final part of the journey, we had to change our focus. When a loved one suffers, you do whatever you can to decrease the hurt of the one you love. Hospice was going to help us with medicines, equipment, and support, all in the context of our home. But Heather would need to be surrounded by love too. Thus, we sought to have as many visitors as she was able to receive, sharing their love, their presence, and their prayers with us.

With Heather lacking energy to write her own posts, our daughter, Kate, took over the duty this time:

> Yesterday my parents met with the hospice nurse and will pursue this avenue next to provide support and care to her. It feels like a hard next step forward, but we have felt God's kindness and goodness to us in this process. My mom has cared for and loved all of us so well, as I know many of you have seen and experienced yourselves, and we feel privileged to care for her now.

Yes, Heather had cared for all of us so well. Now, it was our privilege to care for her—one of the hardest things I have ever done. Thankfully, we were fortified by family, friends, and the presence of God.

For a while, though Heather could eat little, she seemed to rally herself and enjoy the visits. Some were in person, some by video, and some by phone. What was remarkable was that Heather was still Heather, not only sharing about herself but inviting others to share how they were doing.

Thinking back over the last few years, I remembered how on each doctor's visit, they always took out their stethoscopes to listen to her heart, though it was never her heart that was the problem. It made me think now as she listened to others, that Heather had learned how to hear someone's heart without a stethoscope. In her usual way, she said things that helped others. But now there was a special impression she made on them. They were inspired at this point in her life by her demeanor despite her bodily weakness. She was calm and she was caring. She was dying in body; all could see that. As the Scripture says:

> *Though our outer self is wasting away, our inner self is being renewed day by day.*

> *For this light and momentary affliction is preparing us for an eternal weight of glory beyond all comparison, as we look not to the things that are seen but to the things that are unseen. For the things that are seen are transient, but the things that are unseen are eternal.*
>
> **2 Corinthians 4:16-18**

Though Heather remained strong in spirit, I felt weaker in my ability to see the things that are unseen or accept the current affliction as "light." In my internalizing of the stress, I started losing more weight, already a problem given how much I had lost from earlier times when things were hard. Keeping vigil with Heather over these last weeks of her life was going to be a whole-body experience, a physical, mental, and spiritual challenge.

As we crossed into the new year 2023, it felt quite dark as Heather's body shriveled and her energy waned. Now the obstruction was complete, and all she wanted was popsicles. I thought I was helping when I tried to push a little food, but after eating a little and having more pain, I realized I was not helping, but hurting. It was time to give up even the small effort at nutrition and just give the popsicles whenever she asked.

With each day, a further diminishment from the one before, I felt lost, back in Dante's dark wood with no clear way out. I remembered a poem I had heard years before that expressed a way to go forward despite the darkness. Written by Minnie Louise Haskins in 1908, it achieved some notoriety when it was quoted by King George VI in his 1939 Christmas broadcast during World War II. Called *The Gate of the Year*, it felt an appropriate sentiment as 2023 began. In part it reads:

> And I said to the man who stood at the gate of the year:
>
> "Give me a light that I may tread safely into the unknown."
>
> And he replied:
>
> "Go out into the darkness and put your hand into the Hand of God.
>
> That shall be to you better than light and safer than a known way."
>
> So I went forth, and finding the Hand of God, trod gladly into the night.
>
> And He led me towards the hills and the breaking of day in the lone East.

Back in the days when I cared for and walked with many of my uninsured patients outside mainstream health care, I thought I knew something of helplessness as I tried to understand their suffering and pain. But now, walking with my wife as the cancer spread and she wasted away, I was experiencing this powerlessness as never before. When we cannot overcome but only accept and endure, then love must take over, acting in whatever little ways are possible. With darkness all around and no idea of the way to go, it is surely an act of faith to put our hand into the Hand of God and discover that it is better than light or safer than the known way. For me, I saw no other choice. I prayed that somehow, we would make it through.

On January 16, Heather wrote her last post:

These past couple of weeks have been a little intense, and I haven't been very communicative. But when a dear friend asked my family if I was now with the Lord, I realized I need to try and share what is happening.

I was fortunate, for a time, even while already in hospice care, that I was able to eat and drink a bit as the intestinal obstruction caused by the spread of the cancer was still only a partial one. About ten days ago, that changed, and it has now become basically complete …

Sometimes, this is accompanied by pain … Then one night several nights ago, the pain became bigger than me. It felt like the pain was outside my body and was happening to me beyond my control. Pain can be very scary. Thankfully, the night passed, and with Bob's advocacy the next day, the hospice nurses and doctors came to my aid … This is not without God's loving care and spiritual intervention, though! The Lord showed me a promise from Psalm 4:8, "In peace I will both lie down and sleep, for you alone, Lord, make me dwell in safety!" Now, every night as I go to sleep Bob and I pray this prayer and my sleep has been so much more restful … .

In looking back over all the support I have received from you all in these last nearly three years with cancer, I realize that all of the friendships and relationships of my life mattered, and in God's perspective nothing was lost, all is for good. How much I believe your prayers have held me up and protected me. How good God is to love us so well through one another.

Heather's acceptance and endurance and gratitude during these difficult days was a beautiful thing to behold. I felt similar to another spouse walking with her husband over his final days with far-advanced cancer, who wrote, "I had the overwhelming experience of life being enhanced by the acceptance of death." A strange thought indeed, but to see Heather's noble character revealed in these last days will forever enhance my understanding of life.

The days that followed led from one challenge to another as Heather's body kept losing one capability after another. We were regularly in touch with hospice, one day bringing in a shower chair, another day a walker, then the next day a hospital bed. We kept on looking for whatever ways would enhance her life, as diminished as it was. Because until the final hours, her mind stayed strong and her heart caring, allowing her to converse and love all who came to visit.

A few days before her passing, I wrote this post in her CaringBridge journal:

> The light is a lot dimmer at my house this last week. This is Bob, Heather's husband, unfortunately having to write because Heather is just too weak and weary to do it. All of you know of the glimmer in her eyes and the brightness of her smile, now so much diminished in the last few days by pure exhaustion. So, not surprisingly, many of you are not hearing back when you text or write her. Keep texting and writing, because the awareness that

> you are surrounding us with prayers of protection and power make more of a difference than you can possibly realize.
>
> When the body weakens and the spirit wanes to such a high degree, the question comes: When do the blessings of your loved one's presence become a burden unfair to ask them to bear any longer? That time had come for us, to let go and let God.

Four days later, on February 13, my daughter, Kate, spent the day with Heather and me. I thought I might be up most of the night to give Heather whatever medicines might ease her suffering, so I rested in the afternoon while Kate stood watch. About 4 p.m., Kate went home.

And shortly thereafter, at 5 p.m., Heather went home. Kate posted later that night:

> We are gratefully rejoicing that my mom is no longer suffering, having crossed over to the other side tonight around 5 p.m., at peace in the arms of her Savior. This comes one day before my parents would celebrate their thirty-seventh wedding anniversary. We are thankful that in these last days she was surrounded by love, upheld by the support and prayers of those near and far, and in the familiarity of her own home.
>
> We look back on the last three years, thankful for the unexpected time we had with her after her diagnosis, time rich with memories and God's goodness. My mom bore the weight of the physical, emotional, and mental challenges with

> so much grace, clinging to the hope and strength she knew she had in the Lord, and we were so blessed by her. We so treasure the gift of life shared with her … .
>
> We trust that we will see her again, and how sweet that time will be.

At that moment, I had no idea how much I would miss her. I was held together by two consoling thoughts. First, I could not be more relieved that my wife no longer suffered. The last weeks had been hard, and now her journey was over and she was at peace. Secondly, words cannot express how thankful I was that I had been able to fulfill my vows. I had promised when Heather got sick that I would be with her every day, I would never let her suffer alone, and when the time came, I would walk her to the edge of the Jordan and watch her cross over. I saw her go! I knew she had made it! I was there to give her back to God from whom she came. She had always belonged to God. She was never mine. She was given as a gift from God, and for thirty-seven years we lived life together. And now she was returning home, to the place she belonged, with God.

What the philosopher Soren Kierkegaard had inscribed on his tombstone says well what I am sure Heather knew:

> In yet a little while
> I shall have won;
> Then the whole fight
> Will at once be done.
> Then I may rest

> In bowers of roses
> And unceasingly, unceasingly
> Speak with my Jesus.

Challenges to biblical faith

How do you define a premature death?

Many people will colloquially say a person died too soon—and certainly that was said of Heather. I thought it and said it myself.

But when is too soon?

Experts refer to "years of potential life lost"—the number of years a person died before their statistical life expectancy. Some use a standard age, for example, age seventy. By that calculation, Heather died with almost three years of life lost—but that doesn't make sense to anyone who knew her. Overall, she was so healthy and vital that everyone assumed she would live to a much older age.

That's where easy calculations of years of potential life lost break down. Each individual is unique physically and spiritually. Each life is lived in a distinct place and context—and follows a personal path that differs from others.

We need a fuller understanding of whether a person's death is premature, or we are likely to find ourselves adding to our grief with a sense of injustice about when death comes.

Turning to the Bible

Did Heather die a premature death? Statistically, yes. For me as her husband, absolutely.

But by God's standards, I don't think so. By that biblical standard, when Heather died, her work was complete. She had fulfilled her tasks, finished the race, and now had earned the crown of life set aside for her from the foundation of the world.

John the Baptist died in his early thirties, which sounds premature. Yet in the book of Acts, when Paul was speaking of John's ministry that prepared the way for the coming of Jesus, he said that "John was finishing his course" (Acts 13:25). In that way of thinking, it wasn't John's age, but whether he had finished the work he was sent to do that determined whether his death was premature. Paul told Timothy that "the time of my departure has come. I have fought the good fight, I have finished the race, I have kept the faith" (2 Timothy 4:6-7). He was probably about sixty years old when he died, but for him, he had finished the race. Peter similarly saw his time coming, writing that "I know that the putting off of my body will be soon, as our Lord Jesus Christ has made clear to me" (2 Peter 1:14). He was likely in his mid-sixties when he died.

Greatest of all examples is our Lord Jesus Christ. As he approached crucifixion in his early thirties, Jesus knew "that the Father had given all things into his hands, and that he had come from God and was going back to God" (John 13:3). We base our faith upon the completed work of Jesus Christ. He left nothing undone. He accomplished all that the Father had sent him to do. By statistical standards he had many years of potential life lost. From biblical standards, Jesus died when the time was right.

Kierkegaard said we miss this spiritual truth because we believe we have, not numbered days, but days without number. "We keep time with clocks instead of hourglasses," he wrote. "This adds to our delusion, because the hands of a clock go round and round, giving us the impression that our time goes on forever. Hourglasses constantly remind us that for each of us, time is running out."

This is a dramatically countercultural way to think about our lifespan. The Bible teaches us this truth from its earliest passages, calling us to respect the time we have with a reverence that will lead us to consider what we are called to do.

> *So teach us to number our days,*
> *that we may get a heart of wisdom.*
>
> **Psalm 90:12**

> *O Lord, make me know my end,*
> *and what is the measure of my days;*
> *let me know how fleeting I am!*
> *Behold, you have made my days a few handbreadths,*
> *and my lifetime is as nothing before you.*
> *Surely all mankind stands as a mere breath!*
>
> **Psalm 39:4-5**

The Scriptures could not warn us more urgently to be careful with how we keep time. And from these biblical truths flow further awareness of how we are to live. Yes, we should care for our bodies. Our bodies are gifts that should be nurtured—not simply for living long, but for living well.

We seek good health so that we can live faithful lives, so we can run the race with endurance, so that we can "Love God with all our heart and soul and strength and mind" and "Love our neighbor as ourselves."

Despite cultural forces that push against it, the biblical truth is that we discover our purpose within the very frailty and finitude of our physical selves—up to and including the hour of our death. Knowing our days are numbered, we can be wise with the days we have and use them well for the glory of God. And when the time comes, like Heather, and like the many saints of days gone by, we leave this world, saddened for who we leave behind but thankful for having finished the race. For we know our welcome will be great when Jesus presents us "blameless before the presence of his glory with great joy" (Jude 24).

For reflection and discussion

1. Have you been through times when all you could do was sit and be present with a loved one who was dying? In what ways were you able to express love in those difficult days?
2. For those who follow Jesus, we know he has gone to prepare a place for us. Has that truth consoled you as you consider your own death, or helped you to let go when a loved one has passed on?
3. In 2 Corinthians 12:9, in the context of physical disability, God told Paul "My power is made perfect in weakness." What does this mean for you?

4. We all desire to live a full life. What do you think about the idea that completing our journey is less about quantity of time and more about finishing what we were sent to do? Is that comforting? Challenging?

5. What does it mean to number our days? There are websites online that will calculate how many days you've already had since your birth date. Calculate those numbers for the folks in your small group—and you may be surprised at how much time you've had—or may still have ahead of you.

9

A Mystical Union

*This mystery is profound,
and I am saying that it refers to Christ and the church.*
Ephesians 5:32

More than half of Americans are married—and another 20% are in self-defined committed relationships without having taken marriage vows, according to Pew Research. But researchers find it much more difficult to explore what those vows and commitments mean, when people take them. For many of us—and certainly for Heather and me—something more profound than promises "to love and cherish" unfolded when we were married: A mystical union was formed. The theme stretches from Genesis 2 to Jesus' words in the Gospels:

> *A man shall leave his father and mother and hold fast to his wife,
> and the two shall become one flesh.
> So they are no longer two but one flesh.*
> **Mark 10:7-8**

This reality, something Heather and I believed from the start, never became more real than when we walked as one on her journey with cancer. During those three years, I was absorbing a great deal of her pain and suffering within my own body. When she was in pain, I was in distress, and it followed in degrees; if she was in greater pain, then I was in greater distress. When she was having a good day, often so was I. At the most visceral of levels, when Heather didn't feel like eating, neither did I, leading to some significant loss of weight and health on my part. In the first months of her illness, when things were very rocky, I lost over 25 pounds. Many parts of the following year were more stable, and things held steady for a time.

When we entered the last phase of her life, when treatment was over and her abdominal obstruction advanced, she did not feel like eating, and neither did I. We both lost weight. At the time of her death, I had reached my lowest point. In stops and starts I had lost 45 pounds over the three years. When I looked in the mirror, I saw a skeleton looking back. My family and friends were worried about me.

On the day I knelt down to lay the urn with her ashes into the deep hole dug out in the ground, some thought I wouldn't make it back up. I was in a weak and weary state.

What happened to me? Was it because I was internalizing so much stress that my health so badly deteriorated? That certainly played a part. But I think a bigger part was because the two had become one. I could not separate myself from my wife's experience of cancer. It was as if I had cancer, too. Her suffering was my suffering. Her experience in the body was my experience in the body. That is a mysterious reality.

This mystical union, and its subsequent breakage, became a source of significant confusion for me in the first months after Heather's death. Among the many challenges of being alone, I had one very practical concern: After all these years of coping with pain together, who would be with me when I was in pain? Pain hurts, but pain alone is far worse. Over the years, if one of us was ill or in pain, we could talk about how to respond, reassure each other, and even drive to a hospital, if necessary. I feared that day when I would be in pain—and it happened just a few months after Heather died. This was a good day early on, as I went bowling with my son and his family. But by early evening, I began to have pain in my stomach. Still a doctor, I felt like I was thinking clearly when it started, so I tried diagnosing myself. Maybe it was just a passing stomachache. It would eventually let up, I hoped. But the pain did not stop. It only bore more deeply and intensely on the right side of my lower abdomen. With the increasing pain, I soon found myself on the floor curled up in a ball.

I wanted to call out: "Heather, what should I do?"

Or, "Can you take me to the emergency room? I think this is serious."

But Heather wasn't there, and I knew that with the escalating pain my ability to make good decisions was rapidly declining. I called my daughter for some sane thinking about what to do, but she did not answer. Now what? Wait a little longer? See if my next-door neighbor can take me to the hospital? Try calling my daughter again? With the progression of the pain, it was soon obvious she was too far away now to help. I didn't have much time to think. I was afraid I would pass out with the pain.

Something needed to be done. I cried out to God. In my desperation I was even challenging in my tone. "God, you told me to fear not because you would be with me. Well, I am getting afraid and I need you to tell me what to do."

From that moment, every decision I made turned out well. Instead of calling my daughter or my neighbor, I called the ambulance. They arrived quickly but the paramedics were young, inexperienced, and tentative. They started making small talk, clearly unaware of the amount of pain I was having. I told them to take me quickly to the nearest emergency room. When the younger of the two tried to get a needle in my vein and instead hit the artery, blood started spurting everywhere. I told them to stop trying, put pressure where it was needed, and take me to the hospital without delay. It seemed like I was directing the show, something I had never done as a patient before. I was being authoritative but with an authority not my own. For me, I felt the Lord had taken over.

Coming by ambulance instead of by car, I was triaged as needing immediate help and taken to an exam room. The doctor, there within minutes, quickly assessed I was in serious pain and ordered STAT pain medication and a CT scan. Soon the intravenous medication took effect and reduced my pain. The CT scan was done shortly thereafter.

And about an hour later, something surprising happened. My pain simply vanished. From severe pain to no pain at all. How did that happen?

The mystery was soon resolved. The doctor came in with the results of the scan. I had a kidney stone that had gotten stuck, producing a blockage that swelled everything behind it. That accounted for the pain. But its complete disappearance? The only explanation was that the stone had passed, immediately relieving the obstruction.

That night, besides the gift of no longer being in pain, what I remember most was the deep sense I had that I was not alone in my pain. I felt like God was with me, and that most of the choices I made were not because I was smart or had experience as a physician. When you are in pain, you are a patient first and foremost. And people in intense pain, as I have observed as a physician, are not in the best circumstances to make good decisions. They need an advocate, someone who loves them and is there with them. And at that moment for me it was God. It was an answer to my question in the most dramatic terms: "When you are in pain, though Heather is gone, I will be with you."

Later that evening my daughter called back. She wanted to come, but now there was no need. I knew she felt bad that she hadn't been there.

The next day we had an opportunity to talk. I knew she wanted to be there for me as much as I wanted to be there for her. I wanted to fill the hole left by her mother and she wanted to fill the hole left by my wife. But I knew I could not do that for her and she could not do that for me. We both would be an immense support to one another in the days ahead, and to some degree we did help shrink the huge void in our lives left by Heather. But there was a space and a place too deep for either of us to fill for the other.

That hole could only be filled by God.

Challenges to biblical faith

I must admit I struggled greatly with God's ways in marriage after Heather died. How could God make the two into one and then tear them apart? What good purpose could be served by severing that relationship—leaving the other half torn with loose ends flapping in the wind? How can someone who has been made one with another ever be one again when the other half is gone? How could I ever be whole again? I felt like a clay pot pushed off the shelf and broken in pieces on the ground—as in Psalm 31:12: "I have become like a broken vessel."

But God never said marriage is forever. That is the stuff of greeting cards and pop songs. "Endless love," they sing. "Forever together," they write. When we say our vows on our wedding day, we think more about going hand-in-hand through thick and thin together. We forget the time when "death do us part," leaving the other alone.

When death does part us in marriage, if we accept what the world tells us, we can't help but feel that our love has been cut short. But instead of being cheated, what if it actually meant, as C.S. Lewis puts it in *A Grief Observed*: "This had reached its proper perfection. This had become what it had in it to be. Therefore, of course, it would not be prolonged." Or, as Lewis puts it in *Till We Have Faces*: "To love and to lose what we love, are equally things appointed for our nature."

It's hard to think a marriage has reached its completion before we are ready to let it go. But all things have a beginning and an end. Heather and I trusted God on our wedding day. With the engraving of "Phil 1:6" on our rings, we believed that God had begun this marriage and he would bring it to completion. Though it seems unnatural, and though I find it extremely difficult, I want to believe that God completed my marriage to Heather. It had fulfilled its God-ordained purposes. It was whole, it was rich, it was full, and it was complete. And now there must be purpose in the solitary journey I must walk for some time and for some good.

Turning to the Bible

The mystery of the marriage union is talked about perhaps more extensively in Ephesians 5 than anywhere else in the Bible. Here we are asked to love our wives as Christ loved the church and gave himself up for her. Husbands are to love their wives as they love their own bodies. Again, we are reminded that in marriage the two become one flesh. And then the most intriguing statement is made: "This mystery is profound, and I am saying that it refers to Christ and the church" (Ephesians 5:32).

All along we were thinking Paul was talking about the mystery of the marriage bond. But the more mysterious and potent reality is Christ's relationship with those who call him Savior and Lord. That is the relationship above all other relationships and toward which every relationship should aim. In a sense, every other relationship is at its best a likeness of that relationship, an image of the ideal.

As I reflected on my years of being married to Heather, I always knew I was a lucky man. What I received from Heather was the clearest depiction I ever had of God's unconditional love for me. Heather showed me in human form what God's love was like. Imperfect, yes, but truer to the form of the ideal than anything I had ever experienced.

And now God was leading me to the answer to my question. It was God who would make me whole again through the mystery of my union with Christ—an indwelling of Spirit. "I in them and you in me," Jesus prayed on the night before he died, "that they may be perfectly one, so that the world may know that you have sent me and loved them even as you loved me" (John 17:23). For the individual believer, "It is no longer I who live, but Christ who lives in me" (Galatians 2:20). Later John adds richly to this idea in his first letter. God "sent his only Son into the world, so that we might live through him" (1 John 4:9). John also tells us that "we know that we abide in him and he in us, because he has given us of his Spirit" (4:13), and that "God is love, and whoever abides in love abides in God, and God abides in him" (4:16). How beautiful an expression of this mysterious union with God!

Here is where I could find wholeness again. Through my life with Heather, I had been able to see God's love more clearly. And now that Heather was with God, he would be the one through whom I would find wholeness again. Though there was a painful process coming in the months ahead, God already was calling me through my loss toward a deeper relationship.

Suddenly, I saw my sadness and suffering in a new light. God had given us a glowing model of his covenantal love for us in our marriage bond. But the true mystery, as Ephesians 5 describes it, is not the two becoming one in marriage. While that is a great good, the deeper reality is that Jesus Christ has offered us wholeness and oneness in him. With the potential to grow into a deeper life with God, a door slowly began to open for me.

I could look through and see a meaning and purpose for my pain that heretofore was unavailable to me.

For reflection and discussion

1. How do you think about the union of marriage? If you're married, can you describe an example of the "mystical union" of becoming one? What married couple do you know who exemplifies this union?
2. Have you experienced a loss that made you feel as if a part of you was taken from you? In what ways were you able to restore some sense of wholeness over time?
3. What relationships have you had that most reflected the unconditional love of God?
4. How can we let loving relationships in this world draw us toward a more intimate relationship with God?

Stunned

*I will offer to you the sacrifice of thanksgiving,
and call on the name of the Lord.
I will pay my vows to the Lord
in the presence of all the people.*

Psalm 116:17-18

Ever since I knew Heather had incurable cancer, I began anticipating her death.

But anyone who has lost a loved one will tell you: "Will be gone" and "now really gone" are two very different matters. When it finally happens, you are stunned.

First comes numbness and busyness. The numbness, almost an absence of feeling, functions as a survival mechanism as we try to live with the inescapable presence of an inescapable absence. That gives rise to a sense that you are not really here because it is too painful to be aware of where you are. You have been dazed and concussed by a knockout punch that has sent you to the canvas. You are aware that you are not thinking straight, as if your mind has been short-circuited by a tremendous shock.

Having at least the awareness I was not in my right mind, I made sure not to make any major decisions without my daughter, my son, or someone else I trusted to verify it.

Most times, I deferred decisions to others. I just let myself be dazed and bewildered.

And the busyness? Because there was so much to do right away, I was mercifully distracted from the weight of sadness and emptiness. The list of distractions was long:

- The notification of family and friends.
- Making arrangements for cremation, church services, and burial.
- Tending to a myriad of financial details.
- Responding to all the caring people who communicated their love and condolences by visit, by email, and by text.
- Rearranging things in the house for a family of one instead of two.

For a few weeks, these essentials can mask the feelings—but sooner or later a devastating loneliness hits.

The light seems to go out.
The house seems empty.
Inertia sets in.
Even after a full night's sleep, you're exhausted.
Days seem long and repetitive.
Essential tasks seem overwhelming.
Energy evaporates.

I don't know how many of these you've experienced, but I reached a point where I could not wait for night and another chance to escape reality with a little sleep.

A psalm-like prayer by Douglas McKelvey voices that shock so many of us feel:

> Comfort us, O God, in these hard and early hours of our loss.

> Be to us a strength and light, for we are shocked
> and numbed as children spilled into cold seas,
> stunned amidst the sudden wreckage of our ship.

I struggled through each day. Many times, unable to know what to say or do, I took solace in trusting the Holy Spirit would intercede for me "with groanings too deep for words" (Romans 8:26). At first, I thought it best to pitch camp, sit and lie in grief, and sleep away a bit of the delirium. But I knew that it would be dangerous if I stayed too long in the tent I had pitched. I understood there was a great risk of getting stuck, or worse still, sliding into the pit that was already there, the big one right in the center of my being. A bomb had gone off and left a deep crater. It would be so easy to fall in and never get out.

Challenges to biblical faith

One impulse that was very strong in these early months was a desire to escape this world and all the sadness of it. It is a far more common desire than you may think.

As John Donne wrote when he was suffering in the midst of a near fatal case of what was likely typhus in the early seventeenth century: "If man knew the gain of death, the ease of death, he would solicit, he would provoke death to assist him by any hand which he might use ... so when these hourly bells tell me of so many funerals of men like me, it presents, if not a desire that it may, yet a comfort whensoever mine shall come."

Likewise, Dante, in *Vita Nuova*, speaks of where his sorrow drove him on the death of his beloved Beatrice. He weeps until his eyes "were so wept out they could no longer relieve his sadness." Though he accepts at some level her death, he cannot free himself from thinking that his true consolation will only come when he can join her in death. Taken from him by death's cruelty, he is "jealous of whoever dies."

In my grief, I could relate to both Donne and Dante. I wondered if perhaps God would soon take me home, and I actually comforted myself in thinking that might be true. After all, I was already at the lowest physical point I had ever been. And now my emotional and mental states had also reached a nadir. I had just recently been to the metaphorical Jordan River and watched Heather cross over. It seemed a small thing from where I was standing to turn and go back to the river's edge, where I too could wade across.

Turning to the Bible

Of course, I knew I could not count on dying soon, a weak hope at best, and a false one at worst.

At some point, and sooner rather than later, I needed to lift up the sorrow and sadness, heft it onto my back, and start walking—a limping pilgrim carrying a heavy load. I would still return to my little camp and rest in my sorrow from time to time, but the only way to avoid being buried in grief is to get moving.

I thought often of Psalm 23. If I claimed the Lord was my shepherd and if I was his sheep, then I knew I had to get up and get going. I had tethered myself to a sojourning God, one who led the people through the desert, and one who would walk with me through the shadow of death. Yes, we would stop by some green pastures and quiet waters for rest. But what is most important in this image is that God is not only present with us in the darkness, but as a good traveling companion, God encourages us to keep moving along "paths of righteousness" (Psalm 23:3). If we do not keep walking through the darkness, we will sit and we will sink. In obedience to the beckoning of my shepherd, I got up and started going.

Yet after two months, I was still as weak as before, with little appetite for food or life. I had been evaluated by my doctor but there was no medical diagnosis to explain it. Where was I to turn? I desperately needed some measure of healing in mind and body if I was to keep going.

When Easter arrived in April, I knew I was not ready to join a family gathering for the first time without Heather. My sadness could not bear the festivities and reminders such a day would bring. Needing a place to lament, I sought solace along the southern border of the United States. For years, I had been connected to a ministry at the border between El Paso, Texas and Juarez, Mexico called Abara. Their work was concerned with remembering and caring for the pain and struggles of those who have been crossing a particular ford in the river between El Paso and Juarez for centuries—and continue to do so today. They specifically sought to give people a place to lament and a place to heal in the context of human community.

I asked Nate Ledbetter, a friend who was on staff, if I could join him at Abara over the Easter weekend. I asked little—could I be of service? Perhaps wash some dishes or vacuum some rugs? Could I attend a Good Friday service with him? Would he kneel with me at a specific spot on the border where Abara will one day build a chapel for prayer and lament?

He agreed, so for fifteen hours I drove from Denver to the border, seeking a place to weep and a space to heal.

We knelt and prayed on that spot the Saturday before Easter. We prayed for my healing, joining my personal need for bodily and mental renewal with the need for healing for so many others who had suffered in their journey to this same spot over the years. At this unique place at the border, I was participating in grief with a great multitude who had lost so much before getting here. Connecting personal lament with public lament was a powerful conjunction.

This was an unanticipated moment of grace. And when I got home, much to my surprise, I started to eat better. I do not mean to say my pilgrimage to El Paso was akin to those who go to a place like Lourdes and throw away their crutches after some dramatic healing. But for me, it felt like a healing, nonetheless. One month later I was ten pounds heavier, continuing to gain weight with a better appetite, and growing in energy and strength for the things I was trying to do to continue living this life as a follower of Jesus.

In the process of getting back to life, early on I sought to keep it simple, focusing on two practices.

First, I tried to make a commitment to accomplish at least one thing each day. Usually, I would schedule some activity to get me out of the house and meet others who also had needs. I returned to delivering Meals on Wheels, something I had been doing before, Heather often with me when her health allowed. Some days I would serve a meal at a homeless shelter. Or later, when I got healthier, I offered myself as a handyman for the elderly, attaching safety grab bars in the bathroom, changing a light bulb, or fixing a leaky faucet. And eventually I got back to medicine, volunteering as a doctor at a program for the homeless.

Second, I sought relationship and prayer. How true it is that we are never more aware of our need for others than when we hurt. Every day I would try to set up a phone call, video chat, or a visit in person, asking for time to share. I was blessed to have a community of people willing to do this with me. For the first few months, I confined myself to being with people who knew and loved Heather well and would therefore understand my grief. I was determined to be vulnerable with my pain, to be honest with whoever I was with, and ask that each time we would pray before we ended. I cannot express enough how crucial this was in those early days, to avoid isolation and seek supportive community. Many caring friends entered into my grief.

It seemed that the more honest and vulnerable I was, the more blessed others felt to be with me. Somehow true vulnerability is a rare thing that attracts rather than repulses. I do not know how many times I expressed deep gratitude for someone spending time with me, only to be told how much they appreciated being with me. That was a work of the Spirit, I am sure.

Honestly, for much of this time, I did these things as if I was alive but underneath felt like a dead man walking. Unable to feel anything but sadness, with no real motivation for doing anything, I kept telling myself, as my old friends in recovery from alcohol and drugs used to say, just fake it until you make it. You feel as if you are dead, but you have to act as if you are alive.

Whether you like it or not.

Here is where I found myself returning to the wisdom in the second half of Psalm 116—a psalm we began to explore in Chapter 6. When things get murky, we need to return to basics if we are to get moving. Grief is one of those things that makes it very hard to see where you are going. The days seem sunless, gloomy, and dark. All is dim, dull, and overcast.

In the second half of Psalm 116, I found three recommendations about how to keep going that meshed perfectly with the practices I already was trying to adopt.

First, make a commitment and keep it, which is one of those essentials that holds the universe together. Making and keeping vows reflects the covenant-making and covenant-keeping nature of God. There are big vows, like the marriage vow, the vow to raise your children in the faith and direction of the Lord, and the commitment to care for your father and your mother. But everyday there also are opportunities to make much smaller commitments and keep them. Showing up in response to a friend's request for help. Serving on a church or civic committee. Getting to work on time and putting in your best effort throughout the workday. That is why I tried each day to vow to do something—and then do it. It got me going. It got me thinking about something or someone other than myself. And it made me feel I was acting like our covenant-keeping God when I fulfilled my vows.

Second, I see the psalm telling us to bring our thank offerings. One of the great balancers of grief is gratitude. The psalmist knew that God had delivered him from great trouble. I know that God has done the same for me many times in my life. I also knew that having Heather as my wife for thirty-seven years was one of the greatest gifts I could have ever received. One of the surest ways to move through grief is to recall God's faithfulness in the past—and express our thanks for the gifts of life and love already given.

Finally, the psalmist tells us to "call upon the name of the Lord" (verses 13 and 17). Call on God at all times and in all circumstances, both to ask for help as well as praise him for his steadfast love. Constantly reaching out to God for strength, provision, protection, and direction can move the grieving spirit back into the world and once there, engage in it for good.

Make vows and keep them.

Give thanks in all things.

Cry out to God in every situation.

I didn't need to figure out a new way. I needed to return to the basics. That was how I was able get up and get going in my early days of grief.

For reflection and discussion

1. Do you find it hard to be honest and vulnerable with others when you are in pain? Can you describe a time when you found that was a real challenge? How did you resolve that?
2. What does it mean to you to "make vows and keep them" as a daily practice to keep you actively engaged in life?
3. Is "giving thanks in all things" a challenge for you? Have you found that's a useful practice? Do you have any suggestions for how to more regularly express gratitude?

4. And how well do you do in "calling upon the name of the Lord" in times of need? What does that involve for you? And can you share an example?

II

A Thought That Had to Change

> *Where there is true hope, death is approached*
> *not as an occasion for dreaming of an afterlife*
> *but as a task given to me here and now by God:*
> *a claim on my obedience.*
>
> **Glenn Tinder, from The Fabric of Hope**

Many times, I thought my life was over, complete. Perhaps it was time for God to take me home as well.

In the span of my life, I had finished many of the things I felt sent to do. As a physician, I believed that God had called me to serve on the front lines for the underserved and marginalized in health care, and for nearly forty years I had tried to do that both in the United States and internationally. I had been a husband to my wife for thirty-seven years and raised two children, now well-established adults, married with their own children. I walked with my wife step-by-step through three years of cancer and chemotherapy and watched with gratitude and sadness as she safely crossed the Jordan and reached the other side. I felt I had made the vows I was meant to keep and there were no more to make.

I truly had no other goals in life, no bucket list to fulfill, and at a more existential level no reason or sense of meaning for going on without Heather. I did not want to start over. In honesty, I had had enough of this dark and weary world and wanted to escape to heaven and be with Jesus. Never had I been in such complete agreement with the apostle Paul, that "to die is gain" (Philippians 1:21).

I asked God, "Where Heather has gone—may I now come?"

Then one night, about eight months after Heather died, Jesus answered me in a most direct way. In my life, this was the clearest sense I ever had that I was having a conversation with Jesus. Perhaps because of the importance of the message, and how dim and dull I had been to more subtle communication, Jesus saw it was time to speak more clearly.

It was early evening. I was home alone when Jesus spoke to me: "You say that you want to be with me."

"Yes, Lord, I want to be with you."

So far so good. But then came an unexpected and confusing question: "What do you want more: Me or heaven?"

I had been thinking they were one and the same. Now, Jesus surprised me with this stark choice and I had to answer: "You, Lord, I want you."

"Well, if you want me, then stay where you are. Yes, I am present at the right hand of the Father and will remain in heaven until the time comes for my Father to restore everything. But by my Spirit I am in the world. And if you wish to be with me, you will find me in the highways and byways of life, with the poor and needy, and wherever two or three are gathered in my name. If you want me, this is where you will find me and where you can be with me."

I would like to say I was elated to be talking with Jesus. But I must admit that these words were disturbing—a direct challenge to my current understanding of what it meant to be with Christ. In grief and weariness, I wanted to leave the misery and sin of this world behind and thought asking Jesus to take me home was a good thing. In reality, I had been self-indulgently seeking to escape my suffering and grief. Jesus told me I was wrong. I needed to change my thinking and accept that to be close to Christ at this time was to remain right here.

I thought of the passage in John 12, when some Greeks wanted to have an audience with Jesus. They were in Jerusalem to worship at the Passover feast during Jesus' last week on earth. Asking Philip if they could see Jesus, Philip took Andrew and went to present their request. Jesus' response was probably nothing like what they were expecting:

> The hour has come for the Son of Man to be glorified. Truly, truly, I say to you, unless a grain of wheat falls into the earth and dies, it remains alone; but if it dies, it bears much fruit. Whoever loves his life loses it, and whoever hates his life in this world will keep it for eternal life. If anyone serves me, he must follow me; and where I am, there will my servant be also.
>
> *John 12:23-26*

The Greeks, wanting to be with Jesus, thought they might get an easy pass—and that was exactly what I had been looking for!

I thought again and again about that passage from John 12. Jesus asks us to "hate" our life in this world, but that does not mean hating the gift of life itself. What Jesus meant is that we hate the life that keeps us attached to so many things in this world that are distracting us from him and his calling. It means being willing to die to self and follow Jesus, so that "where I am, there will my servant be also."

So, in my conversation with Jesus in that remarkable evening, I finally said, "Okay, Lord, I do want to be with you more than I want to be in heaven. If being with you means being here, I will stay."

I think one of the strongest reasons I believed that I was conversing with God that evening and not just talking to myself was how much this was not the conversation I wanted. Immediately after, I felt deep in my soul how hard this was going to be. But the challenge was clear: I needed to put aside what I wanted in order to be where God wanted me, here and now in union with him.

Of course, I kept talking, hoping for more: "One last thing, Lord. If you can't take me home, then you will have to take over. It is only in your strength that I can do what you are asking."

I did not hear anything after that.

But I think the answer was: I will.

Challenges to biblical faith

Because our culture has done such a good job teaching us that we are in control of our lives, we would like to control the hour of our death as well. We now have a wide range of physical and medical options for prolonging life. But then a day may come when we don't want to delay death but hasten toward it. Tired of this life, we want to end life on our own terms. With the overcoming of legal restraints in many jurisdictions, there is a growing interest in assisted suicide.

Like many of us these days, I have thought about that issue long and hard—and, for me, it is not compatible with my faith in God. Many years ago, I made a decision to give my life to Jesus Christ. If I gave it to him, was I able and willing to take it back? On the evening of my conversation with God, my weak foray into this world's assumptions that I could control the hour of my death was abruptly halted. That was hard to accept when I was so weary of this world. But harder still is denying my faith and taking back control from the One who has walked with me, protected me, and led me through all these years of my life. Why would he stop caring for me now in my hour of greatest need?

I am glad that there are others who have had similar conversations with God. One example is Elijah in 1 Kings 19, who is terrified, exhausted and cries out to God, "It is enough; now, O Lord, take away my life."

Instead, God speaks in a whisper, basically telling Elijah to get up and get going—because God had more for him to do in this world.

Is God saying similar things to me? Might I believe that God still has work for me to do? As a result of my encounter, I have consciously stopped asking God to let me die. Instead of rejecting the life God is giving me, I need to accept it and find ways to affirm it.

Turning to the Bible

For all our days pass away under your wrath;
we bring our years to an end like a sigh.
The years of our life are seventy,
or even by reason of strength eighty;
yet their span is but toil and trouble;
they are soon gone and we fly away. …
So teach us to number our days
that we may get a heart of wisdom. …
Satisfy us in the morning with your steadfast love,
that we may rejoice and be glad all our days.
Make us glad for as many days as you have afflicted us,
and for as many years as we have seen evil.

From Psalm 90

Do you recognize yourself in my dilemma in this chapter? Do you recognize it in the experiences of loved ones or friends? Waiting to die is a sure temptation for those floundering after deep loss. We wonder, "Can these bones live?" (Ezekiel 37:3).

In such times, may we remember the God who we claim as Lord. He is the one who breathes new life into dry bones "and you shall live, and you shall know that I am the Lord" (Ezekiel 37:6).

Kierkegaard had another way of describing the problem of giving up too soon, what he called "The Early Finish."

> When in a written examination the youth are allotted four hours to develop a theme, then it is neither here nor there if an individual student happens to finish before the time is up or uses the

> entire time. Here, therefore, the task is one thing, the time another. But when the time itself is the task, it becomes a fault to finish before the time has transpired. Suppose a man were assigned the task of entertaining himself for an entire day, and he finishes this task of self-entertainment as early as noon; then his celerity would not be meritorious. So also when life constitutes the task. To be finished with life before life has finished with one, is precisely not to have finished the task.

Yes, as the psalmist says, our years are full of toil and trouble. We tire of seeing so much affliction, pain, and evil. But neither the fleeting nature of life, nor the difficulties of living out the fullness of the life you have been given, are an excuse for giving out or giving up. Rather let us be faithful to number our days and count each one as important.

In fact, because of the "steadfast love" of the Lord we can rejoice and be glad. As the psalmist reminds us in the opening verse of this great psalm, the Lord has been "our dwelling place in all generations. Before the mountains were brought forth, or ever you had formed the earth and the world, from everlasting to everlasting you are God."

For reflection and discussion

1. Have you had an experience of God speaking to you? Did you tell other people about it—or keep it to yourself? Can you describe it to friends in your small group?

2. Where are the places you are most likely to see Jesus in your life?
3. Are you in danger—or do you know someone in danger—of dying in spirit before dying in body?
4. How do you number your days? Do you have a daily spiritual discipline, perhaps of reading and prayer? Do you keep a diary or journal? What can you suggest to others about such daily practices?

Collecting Scattered Pieces

*To love at all is to be vulnerable.
Love anything, and your heart will certainly
be wrung and possibly be broken.*

C.S. Lewis from The Four Loves

How did the world become so flat and colorless?

A short time ago, the world was wide and high and deep, brimming with vibrancy and interest and laughter. Suddenly the air rushed out, leaving a deflated and barren land where nothing seemed to matter.

No passion.

No enthusiasm for anything.

Sometimes, I feared that I would never be happy again.

There was that one afternoon, a fleeting moment when I thought I might be feeling happy. Then I questioned if that was appropriate—a foolish thought, for I know Heather would want me to be happy. But the moment quickly passed, and I returned to thinking that without her, happiness was impossible. As Job, I felt as if "my eye will never again see good" (Job 7:7).

I tried simply accepting not being happy. It wasn't my fault. Emptiness and loneliness and sadness dominated the landscape.

Nicholas Wolterstorff, in *Lament for a Son*, put it this way: "I've become an alien in the world, shyly touching it as if it's not mine. I don't belong anymore."

I was glad to see that the psalmist understood, as well:

For my days pass away like smoke, and my bones burn like a furnace.
My heart is struck down like grass and has withered;
I forget to eat my bread.
Because of my loud groaning my bones cling to my flesh.
I am like a desert owl of the wilderness, like an owl of the waste places;
I lie awake;
I am like a lonely sparrow on the housetop.

Psalm 102:3-7

Thousands of years ago, the psalmist was seeing what I was seeing all around me: Smoke. Withered grass. Wilderness. Lonely birds.

I also recalled someone describing the loss of a loved one as if a half-finished jigsaw puzzle is suddenly thrown to the ground. Heather and I enjoyed puzzles during her days of sickness. We would carefully put pieces in place. A pattern would come together. An image would emerge. Then, how terrible to see that table turned upside down—with pieces strewn across the floor. Even as you kneel down, you realize some pieces have slipped under the couch and others have flown who knows where. You pick up the pieces you can find and put them on the table. So many are missing! What is left is unrecognizable from what was there before. Is a new picture possible from the fragments that remain?

That is where much time is spent in the middle of grief, trying to pick up your broken puzzle and put it back together. With that image in mind, this chapter will be a mix of scattered parts and pieces. Or like a bunch of dots on a page that need to be connected but for the moment you cannot see where to draw the lines. Each one has value in and of itself as a way back to wholeness. But how do they connect and where do they fit?

Because I have seen God at work in scattered moments, experiences, conversations, and relationships—I trust one day that I will see them come together into a meaningful whole.

Jerry Sittser, in his helpful book, *A Grace Disguised: How the Soul Grows Through Loss*, describes a transformation in the way he was looking for healing after a devastating loss. His wife, his mother, and his young daughter all died on the same day in a horrible traffic accident. He had a dream where he was frantically running west toward the setting sun, but no matter how fast he ran, the sun just moved farther away until it reached the horizon and vanished. He turned to the east and "saw a vast darkness closing in on me. I was terrified by the darkness. I wanted to keep running after the sun, though I knew it was futile, for it had already proven itself faster than I was." A few days later he shared his dream with his sister. She told him if you want to reach the light, you don't run west toward the setting sun, but turn and run into the darkness that lies to the east—that is the direction where a new day will dawn.

His story reminds me how important it is to enter into the pain and suffering of loss, not run from it. Going through it we will one day see a light dawning in the distance. That hope has guided my path and directed my steps, giving me courage to go through the darkness of grief, not around or away from it.

Accepting that I must walk into the pain of grief if I am ever to come through it, I struggled for many months with how to manage my grief in the healthiest way possible so that I might, one day, see the light dawning again.

Frederick Buechner, the Christian novelist and essayist, lost his father to suicide when he was twelve years old. He had to learn how to live with grief and pain from an early age. In an essay "Adolescence and the Stewardship of Pain" in his book, *The Clown in the Belfry*, he takes the parable of the "talents" in Matthew 25 and turns it on its head. Remember that story? A master is preparing to leave for a while, so he entrusts his property—differing amounts of "talents"—to each servant. One gets five, one gets two, and the third gets one. We generally read the parable assuming the talents are a resource like silver or gold, the most obvious idea, but calling it a talent, perhaps these could have been gifts or abilities. But here Buechner introduces the twist. What if these "talents" are not only about skills or abilities or money? What if these resources that the master is handing over to his servants to manage include pain and suffering?

We all receive differing amounts of suffering in our lives, some much more than others. The question Jesus wants us to ask is not only, "What did I do with my resources and abilities?" but also, "What did I do with my pain and suffering?" Did you steward your pain as well as you stewarded your gifts and abilities? And just as the worst thing you can do with your talents is to bury them, so the worst thing you can do with your pain is to cover it over.

As Buechner goes on to say:

> Bad times happen, good times happen, life itself happens to all of us in different ways and with different mixtures of good and bad, of pain and pleasure, luck and unluck. As I read it, that is what the parable is essentially about, and the question the parable poses is, what do we do with these mixed lives we are given, these hands we are so unequally dealt? ... It is the pain we are given that interests me most here and that I suspect interested Jesus too because God knows he was dealt plenty of it himself during his thirty years on this planet, give or take.

In Jesus' version of the story, the third servant makes the pivotal mistake of taking his pain and hiding it in a hole. He was afraid and he was lazy. He thought he was playing it safe, but he was not really playing at all. Not burying it would be risky, and it would take a lot of work. It is the hardest work of all to grieve well, to live with and through pain and suffering. Burying it never works; it always comes back to haunt you.

The other two servants got it right. They were called "good and faithful." What did they do? They "went and traded with them."

> To trade is to give of what it is that we have in return for what we need, and what we have is essentially what we are, and what we need is essentially each other. The good and faithful servants were not life-buriers. They were life-traders. They did not close themselves off in fear but opened themselves up in risk and hope.

> The trading of joy comes naturally because it is of the nature of joy to proclaim and share itself. Joy cannot contain itself. It overflows. And so it should properly be with pain as well, the parable seems to suggest. We are never more alive to life than when it hurts—never more aware of our own powerlessness to save ourselves and of at least the possibility of a power beyond ourselves to save us and heal us if we can only open ourselves to it.

This challenge of sharing and stewarding our pain for the sake of others gives tremendous hope that our pain and suffering are not in vain.

I saw glimmers of this emerge in my life. Pain is a great motivator, and there were countless days I got out of bed only because if I didn't, I would only get stuck in my pain and feel worse. Then, when I left my house to start another day—to make a vow and keep it—perhaps to enter into the home of an elderly person to help them with their needs—well, then, I realized that I was stewarding my pain for good. This motivation became a piece of the puzzle that I knew would find a central place in the picture that finally would form.

But what picture was that? Of course, I knew the old puzzle Heather and I were putting together was gone. Heather was no longer there. I still was—but I was not the same. Wolterstorff again describes it well, "Something is over. In the deepest levels of my existence something is finished, done. My life is divided into before and after." From now on I carry a load, and a fundamental tone of my life will be sorrow.

Because of my medical training, I was particularly helped by an analogy C.S. Lewis used to describe the trauma of a spouse's death in *A Grief Observed*: "To say the patient is getting over it after an operation for appendicitis is one thing; after he's had his leg amputated it is quite another."

At that time, I thought: I'm the patient Lewis described who loses a leg. I am learning to get about on crutches. Eventually, I will be fitted for a new artificial limb and learn to use it properly. I can still be a pilgrim on the way, a sojourner seeking a better city, but I will get there only by acknowledging that I must adjust to this new way of walking.

Then, after eight months of feeling regularly sad, I began to wonder if something was wrong with me. Shouldn't there have been some relief, some decreased intensity of this sadness by now? I reached out to a missionary friend who had lost her husband six months before Heather died. I asked her to explain what was going on. Of course, she did not try to explain anything, but rather reassured me it was not strange to still feel like I did. She also suggested I join a GriefShare group. This is a Christian ministry that helps churches support people in various stages of significant grief. Joining that group for their thirteen-week curriculum had many benefits, not the least being that I realized I was not abnormal. Praying together, sharing common experiences, and reading various Scripture passages connected to the journey of grief helped immensely.

I realized after that group ended that I had joined a fellowship of grief that I would be bonded to for the rest of my life. I saw that the need to lament is a part of the rhythm of the Christian church—although many men and women who would benefit from this ancient spiritual practice are not finding space for it in their communities of faith. What a wonderful and timely occurrence when my church began a lament-and-praise group around the time my GriefShare group ended. Modeled after the psalms of lament, we would come together and share our longings and our losses—always diligent in following the pattern of Psalms to find ways to praise God in the midst of our sadness.

As I got involved in this circle of people, I found it remarkable how long some people have buried their grief. Becoming an ongoing member of this fellowship of grief and lament, both as a giver and receiver of the comfort therein, became another piece of my puzzle.

Challenges to biblical faith

A great challenge to grieving well is the cultural construct that says we should be strong and get over it. Many people are uncomfortable with sadness, and with being around people who are sad. They often avoid such people, or when with them can only offer efforts, though sincere, to fix the problem. They want your hard times to end, on the one hand because they care, but on the other because they want you to move on so they don't have to deal with your sorrow anymore. Though things are not fine, they want them to be.

I found comfort in thinking of the struggles the prophet Jeremiah faced in his generation. Things were anything but fine in Judah. The people of God had turned from God and were so concerned about themselves that they forgot the needs of those like the sojourner, the fatherless, and the widow, neglecting the covenant. Jeremiah came to tell them that disaster was coming, but the people preferred listening to the "false prophets" who were telling them all was well. One of the most famous passages in Jeremiah is his lament in 6:14: "They have healed the wound of my people lightly, saying, 'Peace, peace,' when there is no peace."

That's how I felt when I encountered people who would ask me how I felt—and I would begin to tell them honestly—only to realize they really did not want to hear my lament. They wanted me to believe that all was well.

Being vulnerable and weak are not common commodities we trade in the marketplace of our culture. They are a hindrance to the cause of high energy, the pursuit of progress, and the optimistic goals we seek to achieve. But the guise of invulnerability will never hold up in the courts of heaven. We are created as dependent and interdependent creatures, made by a God who craves relationship with us. The best thing we can do is avoid the temptation to skim over our grief. May it propel us to meet God in deeper places. Perhaps it may be the first time you ever sought God because until now you never felt you needed him. At last, with the burden so heavy you simply cannot bear it, you are ready to receive Jesus' most wonderful invitation:

> Come to me, all who labor and are heavy laden, and I will give you rest. Take my yoke upon you, and learn from me, for I am gentle and lowly in heart, and you will find rest for your souls. For my yoke is easy and my burden is light.
>
> *Matthew 11:28-30*

Our grief can only be for good if we accept our weakness and vulnerability, refuse to wear masks that say all is well when it is not, and invite God to carry our burdens while asking others to share in our pain. Through such shared vulnerability comes hope for healing and restoration. This was precisely what Jeremiah promised would come to God's people in the future—if they only would face and endure what God had ordained in the present.

Turning to the Bible

I discovered that there were countless ways that Scripture shaped my journey forward and reassured me of God's constant love.

Perhaps my greatest resource, as I turned to the Bible each day, was Psalms—as a starting point to keep going, to keep singing. And in doing so, I realized that I was stepping into the spiritual pathway of so many other pilgrims down through the millennia.

Nicholas Wolterstorff, in *Lament for a Son*, cries out in his anguish: "Are there songs for singing when the light has gone dim?"

And, of course, Leonard Cohen was famous for creating contemporary psalms, the most famous of which is his 1984 *Hallelujah*, which hit such a deep and creative nerve among other artists that it has been rerecorded in more than three hundred versions over the past forty years. What many Cohen fans may have missed, though, was Cohen's 2014 revisiting his classic as he himself kept returning to Psalms. That newer song was called, *You've Got Me Singing* and opens:

> You got me singing
> Even though the news is bad
> You got me singing
> The only song I ever had

And what was that "only song"? At the end of his new song, Cohen sums up his whole life of discovering spiritual renewal in Psalms and psalm-like hymns in three words: "the Hallelujah song."

As I read Psalms, like Cohen, I find comfort and resilience in offering my "broken hallelujah." Many psalms describe a person in desperate circumstances. From there they plead and cry out for God to hear them, to shield them, to deliver them. Usually, as we reach the final verse, we have no reason to believe that the circumstances of the psalmist have changed. Often, as in times of grief, we have no idea when things will change. Yet Psalms render praise and thanks all the same—even in the midst of our darkness—because in those moments of reading or singing, we are taking our eyes off our circumstances to gaze at God. The character of God. The ways of God. The promises of God. The love of God. How God has acted in the past. How God will act in the future.

Consider these treasures from Psalms:

> *The Lord is a stronghold for the oppressed, a stronghold in times of trouble.*
>
> **Psalm 9:9**

*The Lord is my rock and my fortress and my deliverer,
my God, my rock, in whom I take refuge, my shield,
and the horn of my salvation, my stronghold.*

Psalm 18:2

You have seen my affliction; you have known the distress of my soul.

Psalm 31:7

The Lord is near to the brokenhearted and saves the crushed in spirit.

Psalm 34:18

God is our refuge and strength, a very present help in trouble.

Psalm 46:1

*Father of the fatherless and protector of widows is God in
his holy habitation. God settles the solitary in a home.*

Psalm 68:5-6

Blessed be the Lord, who daily bears us up.

Psalm 68:19

*For you, O Lord, are good and forgiving, abounding
in steadfast love to all who call upon him.*

Psalm 86:5

*I know that the Lord will maintain the cause of the
afflicted, and will execute justice for the needy.*

Psalm 140:12

*He gathers the outcasts of Israel, he heals the
brokenhearted and binds up their wounds.*

Psalm 147:2-3

I am overwhelmed, aren't you? Such greatness of love found in One so mighty in power! Truly if we tried to create a God as good as we could make him, we could never approach the actual goodness of God that has been revealed to us in Jesus Christ. Praise God that he is "the exact imprint of his nature" (Hebrews 1:3), who came to earth incarnate and "made him known" (John 1:18).

Looking at Jesus instead of our circumstances invites us to trust in the goodness and greatness of God, even though our own situation remains unchanged. Surely when the psalmist tells us "But let all who take refuge in you rejoice; let them ever sing for joy" (Psalm 5:11), he is not asking us to rejoice because of the dire circumstances that require refuge. It is because we have a place of refuge to go, to a God who is a fortress, who wants to hide us under his wings, be our shield, and give us protection. That is worth singing about.

I came to believe that my life was not over when Heather went home to be with the Lord. I realized that in whatever situation we find ourselves, God always is loving and inviting us forward. I began to see that God's will always includes a vocation—a calling or invitation. And, for me, God's will at the moment was to start a new life without Heather at my side.

To surrender to God's will is never easy. For Jesus in Gethsemane, only with sweat like drops of blood could he say, "Not my will, but yours, be done" (Luke 22:42). For me, this acceptance is as difficult now as it has ever been—and yet now I know: Therein lies the path to peace.

In the third canticle of *The Divine Comedy*, called *Paradise*, the pilgrim Dante, along with his guide Beatrice, arrive at the lowest of the nine heavenly spheres, that of the moon. Here they meet the soul of Piccarda Donati, a kinswoman of Dante's wife. In the course of their conversation, Dante, wondering at the different levels of heaven, asks Piccarda an intriguing question, "But tell me: all you souls so happy here, do you yearn for a higher post in Heaven, to see more, to become more loved by him?"

> She gently smiled, as did the other shades, then came her word so full of happiness, she seemed to glow with the first fire of love. "Brother, the virtue of our heavenly love, tempers our will and makes us want no more than what we have—we thirst for this alone. If we desired to be higher up, then our desires would not be in accord with His will Who assigns us to this sphere; think carefully what love is and you'll see such discord has no place within these rounds, since to be here is to exist in Love. Indeed, the essence of this blessed state is to dwell within His holy will, so that there is no will but one with His; the order of our rank from height to height throughout the realm is pleasing to the realm, as to that King Who wills us to his will."

And then, she utters one of the best-known lines from Dante's masterpiece, "In His will is our peace."

For those caught up in the Love of heaven, there is no desire to be other than where God's will has stationed them. It strikes me that my unhappiness with my current station, if I believe it to be God's will, can only change if I accept it, as Piccarda did, as an act of love. Therein lies the path to peace. Then my peace is not simply in my position but in a person, the one who has assigned me this place in love: "For he himself (Jesus Christ) is our peace" (Ephesians 2:14).

I found that as I began to live in this kind of spiritual reassurance, love was all around me—more than I had ever realized.

I will never forget a woman I had just met through my work with Volunteers of America saying to me: "I love you."

Her sincerity caught me by surprise and, before I could catch myself, I blurted out: "I love you, too."

I was visiting her home in response to her request for help after a fall. I spent the afternoon with her, putting up a handrail so she could walk the fifteen steps down to her basement, and added a grab bar in her shower. We learned about each other's lives in that short afternoon. Though from different races and cultures, we had much in common. She had lived in her house for over forty years and raised her family there, but now lived alone after her husband's death. I told her about the loss of my wife, and as a fellow griever she cried for me.

When I was done, she asked about payment. She was surprised when I told her there was nothing to pay. I was a volunteer. She owed nothing, though she could make a donation if she wished.

When she asked why I did it, I said, "I'm a follower of Jesus. He told me to love God first, and then my neighbor as myself. You are my neighbor—and that is why I am here."

Then she shared about her own faith in the Lord. How beautiful to learn she was my sister in Christ! I had not just helped a neighbor but a member of my family. So, why be surprised that she should love me and that I loved her? It was natural. We were kin.

Somehow this is another piece of the puzzle. When I stop thinking only of who has left us—I begin to see who *is left* among us. There are many to love in this world and be loved by in return. When our loved one dies, love does not stop being the good and wonderful thing that it is. God is love, and when we love, we are like God. Turning myself to the world and continuing to give and receive love are one of the pieces I must fit into the picture.

For reflection and discussion

1. In polls about the Bible, Psalms ranks as the most frequently read book of the Bible. Why do you think that's so?
2. What's your favorite psalm? If you're in a group, consider making a list of your favorites to share with each other.
3. What do you think of Frederick Buechner's idea of "stewardship of pain"?
4. What attributes of God most delight you? How does looking at the goodness of God impact how you view your circumstances?
5. Are there groups in your community like GriefShare that you've found helpful and can recommend to friends?

13

How Long, O Lord?

It is a good thing to learn early that God and suffering are not opposites but rather one and the same thing and necessarily so; for me the idea that God himself suffers is far and away the most convincing piece of Christian doctrine.
Dietrich Bonhoeffer

The longer and deeper you love, the longer and deeper you grieve. Sometimes I wondered if the price of grief was too high, especially on those days when it seemed nothing was changing. Will this darkness, emptiness, and loneliness ever end? Will the weight of grief ever lessen?

Alfred Tennyson wrote, "'Tis better to have loved and lost than never to have loved at all," after the death of his closest friend at twenty-two. I believe that is true; but it does not lessen the pain in knowing it.

"How long, O Lord" is one of the most common cries in Psalms. How long will evil continue to have its way in the world? How long will God see the suffering of the afflicted and do nothing to stop it? How long must your servant wait for your comfort?

Psalm 13 sums it up well:

How long, O Lord?
Will you forget me forever?

> *How long will you hide your face from me?*
> *How long must I take counsel in my soul*
> *and have sorrow in my heart all the day?*

What an intense series of questions to throw before God. How can this psalmist be so bold as to challenge the God of the universe, the Maker of the heavens and the earth, with these demands that God do something and do it soon?

Yet, I am glad the psalmist dared to do so—because those thoughts were mine as well in the apparent hopelessness of deep loss.

Many times, I cried out: "How long, O Lord?"

And the answer I gleaned from Scripture was—"for a little while."

"A little while" are three of the most frustrating and enigmatic words in the Bible. Jesus uses those words to explain in somewhat hazy terms his imminent departure and later return. The disciples are understandably confused.

> Some of his disciples said to one another, "What is this that he says to us, 'A little while, and you will not see me, and again a little while, and you will see me'; and, 'because I am going to the Father'"?
>
> So they were saying, "What does he mean by 'a little while'? We do not know what he is talking about."
>
> Jesus knew that they wanted to ask him, so he said to them, "Is this what you are asking yourselves, what I meant by saying, 'A little while and you will not see me, and again a little while and you will see me'? Truly, truly, I say to you, you will weep

and lament, but the world will rejoice. You will be sorrowful, but your sorrow will turn into joy."
John 16:17-20

The apostle Peter leaves us in much the same place as Jesus when he speaks of "a little while." He promises one day the coming of our salvation "ready to be revealed in the last time. In this you rejoice, though now for a little while, if necessary, you have been grieved by various trials" (1 Peter 1:5-6). Later on, he adds, "And after you have suffered a little while, the God of all grace, who has called you to his eternal glory in Christ, will himself restore, confirm, strengthen, and establish you" (1 Peter 5:10).

To this day, we are puzzled by "a little while," aren't we? That's true at least for anyone who has sunk into the depths of grief. We question when we will see even the first glimmers of dawn that suggest a new day is coming. It is the weight of grief and the wait of grief, a journey with a promise of change up ahead but no idea of when we will turn the corner. We assume that we can endure almost anything if we know how long it will last.

One of the greatest truths I have learned about grief is: We cannot force it into a timeline.

In much of my time of waiting in grief, I felt adrift in the sea with no shoreline visible in any direction. And yet, anyone who knows the sea, knows that its deep waters are always moving—even when the surface seems calm. I came to realize that there were, indeed, powerful currents moving me despite my lack of awareness.

I am in a different place than when this all began. It is not yet a place of happiness or joy. But it is a place of greater rest and peace with what God is doing and will do. I have picked up some old pieces of the puzzle and found that they still fit. I have discovered some new pieces—new friendships, new purposes, new activities. Is a new picture forming? It seems more possible now than before. But there remains the daily battle. Arrayed against me are the many adversaries of my soul—weariness, the weight of sadness, discouragement, and despair—all wanting me to give up. On my side is a God who daily bears me up, takes my burden upon him, and promises to sustain me. I can be glad because God is good.

But the question, "How long, O Lord?" will always be with me.

Isn't this what all of us ask, who live in a broken world groaning for redemption, awaiting Jesus' return when he will reconcile all things in heaven and on earth, bringing justice and righteousness, steadfast love and faithfulness? Yet for now we get no specific answer to our question. Rather, he invites us to share in the divine tension of waiting while the world suffers. "Because the poor are plundered, because the needy groan, I will now arise," God says in Psalm 12:5, yet now is not yet. For "the Lord is not slow to fulfill his promise as some count slowness, but is patient toward you, not wanting that any should perish, but that all should reach repentance" (2 Peter 3:9). When we join with God in his patience and forbearance, we wait.

We don't know how long "a little while" is. All he promises is that it will not be too long.

Challenges to biblical faith

The book of Job is not easily read in our day and age. A man loses everything—his possessions, his children, and finally his health—and is left to figure out where God is in the midst of so much suffering. The words of Job 5:7 "But man is born to trouble as sparks fly upward" are surely disorienting to our modern sensibilities. Our culture has no time for such pessimism.

We want to live forever and, if we can't, then we at least want to enjoy ourselves here as long as possible. Our modern mentality is that suffering is a problem to be fixed. In such a culture, suffering becomes meaningless, an absurdity inhibiting our autonomy.

Yet only a culture that admits the essential role of suffering as a part of human life can be truly helpful to those who suffer. A culture that perceives all pain and suffering as avoidable or curable makes any pain or suffering intolerable and purposeless. That kind of mentality contributed to our recent opioid crises. What we created was innumerable people addicted to prescription drugs and countless others who died of overdoses with these drugs. How miserably our culture failed to teach people that some suffering and pain is inevitable in our lives.

The Bible has a very different story to tell about pain and suffering and the need for patient endurance. Countless times we are told of our need to wait even in the midst of our suffering. Waiting is a central theme in Psalms.

> *Wait for the Lord;*
> *be strong, and let your heart take courage;*
> *wait for the Lord!*
>
> **Psalm 27:14**
>
> *Our soul waits for the Lord; he is our help and our shield.*
>
> **Psalm 33:20**
>
> *Be still before the Lord and wait patiently for him.*
>
> **Psalm 37:7**
>
> *For God alone my souls waits in silence; from him comes my salvation.*
>
> **Psalm 62:1**
>
> *I wait for the Lord, my soul waits, and in his word I hope;*
> *my soul waits for the Lord more than watchmen for the*
> *morning, more than watchmen for the morning.*
>
> **Psalm 130:5-6**

The biblical witness recognizes the difficulty of waiting. In Romans 8:18, we read that, while our sufferings are for a little while, they are "not worth comparing with the glory that is to be revealed to us." The book of James uses multiple examples to illustrate: a farmer waiting for his crop, the suffering and patience of the prophets who spoke in the name of the Lord, or the steadfastness of Job. Be patient, be patient, be patient, we are told over and over. "Patiently endure the same sufferings that we suffer," Paul advises his readers in 2 Corinthians 1:6. The apostle John considers us brothers and partners "in the tribulation and the kingdom and the patient endurance that are in Jesus" (Revelation 1:9).

These exhortations are a rock in the river of the cultural currents that surround us. And I am not alone in pointing out this huge conflict with our prevailing culture. Especially as he became increasingly aware of his own physical demise, Pope Francis wrote, preached, and taught extensively about our Christian awareness and response to suffering. In February 2025, in a letter to the world he wrote:

> More than anything else, suffering makes us aware that hope comes from the Lord. It is thus, first and foremost, a gift to be received and cultivated, by remaining "faithful to the faithfulness of God." Indeed, only in Christ's resurrection does our own life and destiny find its place within the infinite horizon of eternity. In Jesus' paschal mystery alone do we attain the certainty that "neither death, nor life, nor angels, nor rulers, nor things present, nor things to come, nor powers, nor height, nor depth, nor anything else in all creation, will be able to separate us from the love of God" (Romans 8:38-39).

Like Francis in his extensive writings on suffering, I have always found it comforting to realize that Jesus took the form not of a triumphant superhero—but of a suffering servant. For Christians, Isaiah foreshadows that our coming Messiah would be a "man of sorrows and acquainted with grief" (Isaiah 53:3). Suffering is so central to the nature of Christ that Matthew set aside the better part of the last eight of the twenty-eight chapters of his Gospel, Mark devoted the last six of sixteen chapters, Luke used the last five of twenty-four chapters, and John, most of all, reserved ten of twenty-one chapters to describe the last week of Jesus' life. All that attention given to that one week reveals how important was the Passion of Jesus Christ, including his arrest, suffering, and death by crucifixion. That Jesus Christ suffered, died, and rose again is critical for our salvation. But it is also essential to the way we live out our faith—and can completely change our perspective on suffering.

Since "a disciple is not above his teacher, nor a servant above his master" (Matthew 10:24), if our Lord suffered, then we should expect no less. This will not be easy. Just as his first followers had the greatest difficulty accepting that they were following a suffering Lord, so will we.

At the same time, we also need to be clear: Suffering is not our goal or desire. Jesus did not first and foremost choose to suffer. He chose to be obedient to the will of his Father. That obedience led to his suffering. Our obedience will likewise lead to our suffering. But it is not suffering that we seek. We seek to be followers of Jesus—and Jesus leads us toward compassionate care for all those who are suffering. If we are truly living out our Christian calling, our lives are likely to be surrounded by suffering.

But, in the midst of our own suffering—and in our ministry to help alleviate the suffering of others, as Francis repeatedly proclaims: We will discover more of God's grace in our own lives. In his February 2025 letter, he put it this way: "God does not abandon us and often amazes us by granting us a strength that we never expected and would never have found on our own."

Turning to the Bible

My God, My God, why have you forsaken me?
Why are you so far from saving me, from the words of my
groaning? O my God, I cry by day, but you do not answer,
and by night, but I find no rest.

Psalm 22:1-2

When I read these words during some of the darkest times, I felt they expressed my experience better than any of my own words could express. While most of the Bible speaks *to* us, the Psalms speak *for* us.

I found great hope in realizing that humans have been calling out to God like this through all ages—and, as a Christian, I find great hope in this passage because of its Messianic foreshadowing that points me always toward my hope in Christ. Verses 6-8, for example, describe someone who will be "scorned by mankind and despised by the people. All who see me mock me; they make mouths at me; they wag their heads." As I read such a passage, I am reminded of the suffering and death of Jesus Christ. And, I am reminded that Christ's suffering will always be greater than any I will ever experience.

Whatever depth of suffering we may endure in our lives, Christ's suffering stands beneath it. More deeply downtrodden than anyone will ever be, it places him under us, and thus able to hold us up no matter how low we go. This has been a source of great hope for me. When I feel I am falling headlong into the abyss of my grief, I will never reach bottom, because before I get there, I will be caught in the arms of Jesus Christ standing under me in his suffering.

How reassuring to know that God never turns away from us in our suffering. Quite the contrary, "he has not despised or abhorred the affliction of the afflicted, and he has not hidden his face from him, but has heard, when he cried to him" (Psalm 22:24). No matter how far down, depressed, and immobile we are in our grief, it never offends God.

Psalm 31:7 tells us: "I will rejoice and be glad in your steadfast love, for you have seen my affliction; you have known the distress of my soul."

How truly wonderful that we have a God who is "near to the brokenhearted and saves the crushed in spirit" (Psalm 34:18).

I don't know how many times I told God, "You must be very close, Lord, because I am very brokenhearted."

That Christ suffered to a depth greater than any other sufferer will ever bear—and that God draws close to us and bears us up in our grief—are firm realities of our faith that can carry us through the deepest valleys we will ever face.

For reflection and discussion

1. Where do you encounter suffering? In your own life? Your family? Your neighborhood or place of work?
2. What helps you to endure? What inspires you to service?
3. More than fifty million Americans are daily caregivers among family and friends—and some studies estimate that number may be as high as one hundred million, depending on the definition of "caregiving." That means your workplace, your neighborhood, and your congregation all include many full-time caregivers. Encourage

these folks to tell their stories of service. What can you tell others about your experience with caregiving?

4. What strengths and challenges have you encountered as a caregiver?

14

Embracing God's *Chesed*

*He became what we are
that we might become what he is.*

St. Athanasius

In this final chapter, I humbly offer you two words that I hope will be blessings in your journey through grief: *chesed* and *theosis*.

No, I am not saying that your grief will end, because I hope I have convinced you that grief is not a problem to be solved—but an experience to integrate into our souls. The deepest losses in life will be a part of us for as long as we live. As Nicholas Wolterstorff beautifully explains it in his memoir of wrestling with the grief of losing his son:

> So shall I struggle to live the reality of Christ's rising and death's dying. In my living, my son's dying will not be the last word. But as I rise up, I bear the wounds of his death. My rising does not remove them. They mark me. If you want to know who I am, put your hand in.

So, how do we move forward, carrying our wounds with us? All I can tell you in this final chapter is that these two words—*chesed* and *theosis*—capture truths that have helped me to continue my journey.

Chesed is one of the loveliest words in the Bible—translated by Rabbi Lenore Bohm in her new guide to Genesis as "kindness, graciousness, faithfulness, and lovingkindness." Ancient rabbis regarded *chesed* as the core ethical value in Torah, the first five books of the Bible—God's unfathomable, unfailing, and unending love for us and God's call for us to embody that lovingkindness to others. It is a completely undeserved kindness and generosity, the actions of God based on covenant and promise, unrelated to the worthiness of the recipient.

God, in *chesed*, responds to us in practical actions on our behalf. He rescues us, he delivers us, he saves us because of *chesed*. In Exodus 34:6, we see it is one of the primary attributes of God. As the Lord comes down in the cloud, he stands with Moses and proclaims his name, "The Lord, the Lord, a God merciful and gracious, slow to anger, and abounding in *chesed* and faithfulness." When God liberates Israel by the parting of the Red Sea, the song Moses and Miriam sing is of a God who keeps his promises, who has "led in your *chesed* the people whom you have redeemed" (Exodus 15:13). It is a permanent posture of God toward us, as the prophet Isaiah wrote, "For the mountains may depart and the hills be removed, but my *chesed* shall not depart from you, and my covenant of peace shall not be removed" (Isaiah 54:10).

This vital and vibrant word is used hundreds of times in the Hebrew Scriptures. It is the heartbeat of Psalms, the prayer book of the Bible, where it is found more than in any other Old Testament book. In Psalm 90, that pillar among the psalms that we explored earlier, the psalmist declares that it is only because of God's *chesed* that we can hope to continue.

> *Satisfy us in the morning with your chesed,*
> *That we may rejoice and be glad all our days.*

Psalm 90:14

The New Testament, originally written in Greek, often finds Greek equivalents for the Hebrew term—words like *eleos* and *agape* that capture this concept of merciful love. Think of New Testament stories like the Good Samaritan, the Prodigal Son's father, or Jesus weeping over Jerusalem. These are pictures of *chesed* in motion.

When our circumstances are heavy with grief and sorrow, when the life we are living seems too much to bear, we can claim with the psalmist that God's *chesed* is better than life (Psalm 63:3). It can help us to stand up against whatever trouble or affliction lies in our path—and for however long they last.

The other term—*theosis*—is Greek and offers an astounding possibility: that we might be "made like God," that we may become holy in our life with Christ, that we may become "partakers of the divine nature" (2 Peter 1:4).

It's a term common in Eastern Orthodox Christianity, where the mystical tradition played a stronger role in theology than in the West's more intellectual Christian history. Of course, both traditions produced great scholars as well as mystics—and the message of this book is that we need both. My very act of writing this book—and your reading of it—is an exercise in learning intellectually about stages of grief. Discussing this book with others is also a mutual learning experience that builds healthy community among us. But I have also been pointing you toward deeper spiritual disciplines in your own life—and to considering the leaps of faith that I found so helpful in my own journey. I even shared with you in these pages my own mystical experience of a fleeting conversation with Jesus.

The offer of *theosis* reflects God's intention from the moment of our redemption that "as he who called you is holy, you also be holy in all your conduct, since it is written, 'You shall be holy, for I am holy'" (1 Peter 1:15-16). The book of Hebrews offers a most tender expression of this call to holiness: "For he who sanctifies and those who are sanctified all have one source. That is why he (Jesus) is not ashamed to call them brothers and sisters" (Hebrews 2:11). We are siblings, members of the family of Jesus Christ. Jesus became like us, that we might become like Jesus.

This calling is great yet let us never naively assume it is easy. That's what C.S. Lewis tells us in *Mere Christianity*: "The command 'Be ye perfect' is not idealistic gas. Nor is it a command to do the impossible. He is going to make us into creatures that can obey that command. ... The process will be long and in parts very painful, but that is what we are in for. Nothing less."

It is reassuring to know this process depends more on God and less on us. Our job is to behold God. As 2 Corinthians 3:18 tells us, God will do the transforming work: "And we all, with unveiled faces, beholding the glory of the Lord, are being transformed into the same image from one degree of glory to another. For this comes from the Lord who is the Spirit."

As "those who are being sanctified" (Hebrews 10:14), we are on a life-long journey of growth in godliness. Often connected to our pain and suffering, this understanding can impart great hope that deep meaning and purpose lies within God's companionship in our grief.

There are several ways that our grief and pain can help to carry us along the path toward *theosis*—becoming like God. First, by virtue of the nature of profound loss, many of the physical, mental, and emotional certainties that we had heretofore depended on are gone. Thus, we are forced to throw ourselves into the arms of God as never before. No longer having the luxury to drift along, we become desperate for God's presence.

> *O God, you are my God; earnestly I seek you;*
> *my soul thirsts for you, my flesh faints for you,*
> *as in a dry and weary land where there is no water*
>
> **Psalm 63:1**

Second, our vulnerability made blatantly bare by our loss makes us more sensitive to the vulnerability, pain, and suffering of others. How much like God we become when we care about the broken-hearted and want to help those disheartened, downcast, and discouraged by life's troubles and afflictions.

Finally, our hurting heart may more easily feel the pain of our world in a more cosmic sense—once again identifying with the heart of God who mourns for the brokenness around us.

In my own grief, I often pondered the biblical stories from the time God's people were forcibly dislocated to Babylon—an unfamiliar land, foreign in every way. They do not like the customs, language, music, or foods. They long to return to their home. Making matters worse are false prophets telling them not to worry, because the exile soon will end. Then, in the middle of these false assurances comes the rebuke of the prophet Jeremiah, who was still in Jerusalem. I am sure that this message shocked them to no end. Instead of telling God's people that this sojourn would not be long—Jeremiah told them they should settle in for a long haul. Eventually, God would faithfully lead them home—but meanwhile they should build houses, plant gardens, have children and, in other words, get on with daily living. Even more, "seek the welfare of the city where I have sent you into exile, and pray to the Lord on its behalf, for in its welfare you will find your welfare" (Jeremiah 29:7).

Of course, from our perspective looking across the breadth and depth of the Bible, we recognize Jeremiah's wisdom—and we realize that the people of God have known this truth for a long, long time. After all, it was Moses himself who, in Exodus 2, named his first son Gershom, often translated: "I am a stranger in a strange land."

As I experience life without my wife of thirty-seven years, I feel much like Moses, Gershom, and Jeremiah. I have my house—but I no longer call it "home." Although I feel more than ever the foreignness of life in this world—though I long for the city that is to come as never before—I know that God is calling me now to seek the peace and prosperity of the city where I now dwell.

And in so doing, I find myself more easily able to identify with others who are dislocated and homeless. That identification has opened my heart to all who wander the face of this globe as refugees. According to the United Nations

Commissioner for Refugees, more people have been forced to flee their homes than ever before, with a staggering 110 million individuals displaced worldwide. My sense of personal dislocation gives me greater compassion for the dislocation that so many experience today. I know that this calling is *theosis*—moving closer to the heart of God, who grieves for the wanderer without a home and longs to bring solace to the lonely and the suffering.

This then is the great possibility that lies before those of us who grieve—that we might mourn the very things God mourns. It is one possible sign of life from death, that we who are made in the image of God now mirror God in his *chesed* for the world's suffering.

We now see the world as we never have before. As Wolterstorff describes it:

> Standing on a hill in Galilee, Jesus said to his disciples: Blessed are those who mourn, for they shall be comforted. … Why cheer tears? It must be that mourning is also a quality of character that belongs to the life of his realm. Who then are the mourners? The mourners are those who have caught a glimpse of God's new day, who ache with all their being for that day's coming. … They are the ones who realize that in God's realm no one is hungry and who ache whenever they see someone starving. … They are the ones who realize in God's realm there is no one who suffers oppression and who ache whenever they see someone beat down.

As we wake up every morning on our journey of grief and grace, we wonder where we belong. Whether we see ourselves in the barrenness of the Exodus wilderness or the foreignness of the Babylonian exile, we have a choice of surrendering to our fears—or leaning into our relationship with God. In faith, we can say: "Blessed be the Lord, who daily bears us up" (Psalm 68:19). In comfort, we know: "This I know, that God is for me" (Psalm 56:9). And in hope, we can say: "From the depths of the earth, you will bring me up again" (Psalm 71:20).

We who are in Christ are truly blessed on our journey of grief.

Never alone.

Always loved.

Daily guided.

And so I say to you:

Go and remember the hope of *chesed* and *theosis*!

May you live always in God's steadfast love—and may your journey lead you, each day, closer and closer to God.

For reflection and discussion

1. When have you felt like a stranger in a strange land?
2. What are some of your favorite Bible passages illustrating God's steadfast love?
3. How does your awareness of God's *chesed* shape your own responses to the world's needy people?

4. What do you think of this journey of *theosis*? Are there ways you see that playing out in your own life? Are there people you regard as spiritual mentors who might embody aspects of *theosis*?
5. Are there passages from this book that you would like to share with family and friends?

Finding Solace in Scripture

Throughout this book, I point readers to portions of Scripture that can help in the long journey of sickness, suffering, death, and grief. I am adding this final section as a summary of helpful starting places in Scripture. If any of these verses seem helpful, I encourage you to open your Bible—or your Bible app on your phone or tablet—and read the entire portion. These verses are intended as convenient bookmarks to quickly find passages that may speak to your heart and soul in this journey. They're also great starting points to spark discussions with friends or in a class or small group. (These quotations are from New Revised Standard Version Updated Edition—NRSVue—compiled by a team of fifty Bible scholars and first released online in 2021.)

In darkness and desperation

Turn to me and be gracious to me, for I am lonely and afflicted. **Psalm 25:16**

Be gracious to me, O Lord, for I am in distress; my eye wastes away from grief, my soul and body also. **Psalm 31:9**

As a deer longs for flowing streams, so my soul longs for you, O God. **Psalm 42:1**

Rouse yourself! Why do you sleep, O Lord? Awake, do not cast us off forever! Why do you hide your face? Why do you forget our affliction and oppression? **Psalm 44:23-24**

Fear and trembling come upon me, and horror overwhelms me. And I say, "O that I had wings like a dove! I would fly away and be at rest." **Psalm 55:5-6**

Save me, O God, for the waters have come up to my neck. **Psalm 69:1**

In the day of my trouble I seek the Lord; in the night my hand is stretched out without wearying; my soul refuses to be comforted. **Psalm 77:2**

O Lord, God of my salvation, at night, when I cry out before you, let my prayer come before you; incline your ear to my cry. **Psalm 88:1-2**

I am like a desert owl of the wilderness, like a little owl of the waste places. I lie awake; I am like a lonely bird on the housetop. **Psalm 102:6-7**

How long must your servant endure? **Psalm 119:84**

Out of the depths I cry to you, O Lord. **Psalm 130:1**

Answer me quickly, O Lord; my spirit fails. Do not hide your face from me, or I shall be like those who go down to the pit. **Psalm 143:7**

Chesed—the steadfast love of God

But I trusted in your steadfast love; my heart shall rejoice in your salvation. I will sing to the Lord, because he has dealt bountifully with me. **Psalm 13:5-6**

Steadfast love surrounds those who trust in the Lord. **Psalm 32:10**

He loves righteousness and justice; the earth is full of the steadfast love of the Lord. **Psalm 33:5**

O my strength, I will watch for you, for you, O God, are my fortress. My God in his steadfast love will meet me. **Psalm 59:9-10**

Because your steadfast love is better than life, my lips will praise you. **Psalm 63:3**

When I thought, "My foot is slipping," your steadfast love, O Lord, held me up. When the cares of my heart are many, your consolations cheer my soul. **Psalm 94:18-19**

For as the heavens are high above the earth, so great is his steadfast love toward those who fear him. **Psalm 103:11**

For his steadfast love endures forever. (A refrain repeated in all 26 verses of **Psalm 136**.)

Let me hear of your steadfast love in the morning, for in you I put my trust. **Psalm 143:8**

The steadfast love of the Lord never ceases; his mercies never come to an end; they are new every morning; great is your faithfulness. **Lamentations 3:22-23**

Hope in the midst of suffering and death

When the righteous cry for help, the Lord hears and rescues them from all their troubles. The Lord is near to the brokenhearted and saves the crushed in spirit. **Psalm 34:17-18**

Cast your burden on the Lord, and he will sustain you; he will never permit the righteous to be moved. **Psalm 55:22**

You have kept count of my tossings; put my tears in your bottle. Are they not in your record? **Psalm 56:8**

Whom have I in heaven but you? And there is nothing on earth that I desire other than you. My flesh and my heart may fail, but God is the strength of my heart and my portion forever. **Psalm 73:25-26**

Return, O my soul, to your rest; for the Lord has dealt bountifully with you. For you have delivered my soul from death, my eyes from tears, my feet from stumbling. **Psalm 116:7-8**

Those who go out weeping, bearing the seed for sowing, shall come home with shouts of joy, carrying their sheaves. **Psalm 126:6**

The Lord is faithful in all his words and gracious in all his deeds. The Lord upholds all who are falling and raises up all who are bowed down. **Psalm 145:13-14**

He heals the brokenhearted and binds up their wounds. **Psalm 147:3**

Do not fear, for I am with you; do not be afraid, for I am your God. **Isaiah 41:10**

I will turn the darkness before them into light, the rough places into level ground. **Isaiah 42:16**

The spirit of the Lord God is upon me because the Lord has anointed me; he has sent me to bring good news to the oppressed, to bind up the brokenhearted. **Isaiah 61:1**

Likewise the Spirit helps us in our weakness, for we do not know how to pray as we ought, but that very Spirit intercedes with groanings too deep for words. **Romans 8:26**

For in him every one of God's promises is a "Yes." **2 Corinthians 1:20**

Praise in the midst of grief

I keep the Lord always before me; because he is at my right hand, I shall not be moved. Therefore my heart is glad, and my soul rejoices; my body also dwells secure. **Psalm 16:8-9**

I call upon the Lord, who is worthy to be praised, so shall I be saved from my enemies. **Psalm 18:3**

But may all who seek you rejoice and be glad in you; may those who love your salvation say continually, "Great is the Lord!" **Psalm 40:16**

Blessed be the Lord, who daily bears us up; God is our salvation. Our God is a God of salvation, and to God, the Lord, belongs escape from death. **Psalm 68:19-20**

Happy are those who know the festal shout, who walk, O Lord, in the light of your countenance, they exult in your name all the day, and extol your righteousness. **Psalm 89:15-16**

O come, let us worship and bow down; let us kneel before the Lord, our Maker! For he is our God, and we are the people of his pasture, and the sheep of his hand. **Psalm 95:6-7**

Sing to him, sing praises to him; tell of all his wonderful works. Glory in his holy name; let the hearts of those who seek the Lord rejoice! Seek the Lord and his strength; seek his presence continually. **Psalm 105:2-4**

Praise the Lord, for the Lord is good; sing to his name, for he is gracious. **Psalm 135:3**

Helpful perspectives

I will instruct you and teach you the way you should go; I will counsel you with my eye upon you. **Psalm 32:8**

Why are you cast down, O my soul, and why are you disquieted within me? Hope in God; for I shall again praise him, my help and my God. **Psalm 42:5-6**

Be still and know that I am God! I am exalted among the nations, I am exalted in the earth. **Psalm 46:10**

This is God, our God forever and ever. He will be our guide forever. **Psalm 48:14**

Lord, you have been our dwelling place in all generations. Before the mountains were brought forth or ever you had formed the earth and the world, from everlasting to everlasting you are God. **Psalm 90:1-2**

You who live in the shelter of the Most High, who abide in the shadow of the Almighty, will say to the Lord, "My refuge and my fortress, my God, in whom I trust." **Psalm 91:1-2**

If it had not been the Lord who was on our side—let Israel say—if it had not been the Lord who was on our side … then the flood would have swept us away, the torrent would have gone over us; then over us would have gone the raging waters. **Psalm 124:1-2, 4-5**

O Lord, my heart is not lifted up; my eyes are not raised too high; I do not occupy myself with things too great and too marvelous for me. But I have calmed and quieted my soul, like a weaned child with its mother. **Psalm 131:1-2**

The Lord will fulfill his purpose for me; your steadfast love, O Lord, endures forever. Do not forsake the work of your hands. **Psalm 138:8**

I have said this to you so that in me you may have peace. In the world you face persecution, but take courage: I have conquered the world. **John 16:33**

And not only that, but we also boast in our afflictions, knowing that affliction produces endurance, and endurance produces character, and character produces hope, and hope does not put us to shame, because God's love has been poured into our hearts through the Holy Spirit that has been given to us. **Romans 5:3-6**

Blessed be the God and Father of our Lord Jesus Christ, the Father of mercies and God of all consolation, who consoles us in all our affliction, so that we may be able to console those who are in any affliction, with the consolation with which we ourselves are consoled by God. **2 Corinthians 1:3-4**

So we do not lose heart. Even though our outer nature is wasting away, our inner nature is being renewed day by day. For this slight, momentary affliction is producing for us an eternal weight of glory beyond all measure, because we look not at what can be seen but at what cannot be seen. **2 Corinthians 4:16-18**

Therefore, let those suffering in accordance with God's will entrust their lives to a faithful Creator, while continuing to do good. **1 Peter 4:19**

Additional Support and Further Reading

GriefShare

This 12-week program, offered nationwide at many locations in each region, provides a sensitive, caring, and instructive environment for processing grief. Knowing there are others who are walking the same path, and having wise voices who can encourage you to continue on the way with hope, is an invaluable resource. You can find groups meeting in your area at: GriefShare.org

CaringBridge

One of the most important sources of consolation when you are travelling on a journey of sickness is the support of community. CaringBridge is a very useful, centralized way to communicate with your friends and loved ones. It's simple to set up your own webpage at CaringBridge.org. Visitors to the nonprofit's website will find this description: "CaringBridge is a trusted place to communicate to your community, capture your thoughts and coordinate help on your terms."

Books

There are many books that can help you process the pain of loss and the need for letting go that is inherent in sickness and death. In no way attempting to offer a comprehensive list, let me suggest a few books that have helped me understand and accept the reality of great loss:

Nicholas Wolterstorff, *Lament for a Son*. Beautifully written, this book explores the depth of grief after the loss of a son. The poignancy with which the author describes his feelings invites readers to enter into their own painful places and find hope and love.

C.S. Lewis, *A Grief Observed*. A classic book in the world of grief, Lewis describes his struggle to survive after the death of his wife.

Douglas McKelvey, *Every Holy Moment, Volume II: Death, Grief, and Hope*. A book of short readings and liturgies grouped according to different seasons of dying and grieving. For personal use or as a part of a church service.

Jerry Sittser, *A Grace Disguised*. Another classic written by a professor of theology whose wife, mother, and daughter all died on the same day in a horrific car accident. His thoughtful description of his path toward healing has been a blessing to many.

Joseph Cardinal Bernadin, *The Gift of Peace*. Finished just before his death, Cardinal Bernadin reflects on the last three years of his life and the calm and peace he felt as he approached his imminent death.

Brother Lawrence, *The Practice of the Presence of God*. Not a book about grief, but a series of meditations about knowing and loving God in every hour of every day. For nearly three hundred years, it has blessed and instructed many in the path of peace.

Acknowledgments

Journaling as a way of processing your grief can be an extremely helpful exercise. Writing when you don't want to write—but having people around you insisting that you have something to say—is a whole other story. In the midst of numbing grief it is an overwhelming task, one you could never bear on your own. It is only because of the encouragement and prayers of many people that I sat down and believed that what I might say could be a witness to the faithful life of my wife, Heather, and an opportunity to glorify God for his steadfast love.

First and foremost, it was our children, Kate and Steve, who saw that what I was writing might be a blessing to others. They read what I wrote, contributed their invaluable perspectives on the journey, and confidently encouraged me to push forward to write and seek to publish this work. Kate has also contributed her unique perspective as her mother's daughter in the foreword. Her voice, the voice of a child's loss, is important to hear. I am also thankful for the

Acknowledgments

contribution of my daughter-in-law, Rachel, whose careful look at the final document helped reassure me that we had done our best.

My dear friend, Steve Ridge, has walked closely with me on this journey of loss. We met in church on a Sunday in the summer in 2023, and from that day forward have shared in the fellowship of grief. His loss of his wife, Barb, less than two months before Heather's death, bonded us in a common desire to cling to God in the midst of our sadness. His support of this book has been unflagging from the moment I told him I was attempting such an endeavor. I will always be grateful that God brought us together at just the right time.

Mark and Pam Semmler were the closest of friends to Heather and I, both before she got sick and more closely thereafter. Their ability to be present in every circumstance, to rejoice with those who rejoice and mourn with those who mourn, represents their deep love of God and others. They prayed with me through every step of this effort to write something that would be a true representation of God's grace and mercy for people in pain.

Dave and Jennifer Erickson have loved Heather and me for a very long time. They came so close to us when Heather got sick, and their unwavering presence, their total commitment to prayer, and their continued support to me after Heather died have uplifted and sustained me on many occasions.

I am grateful to the physicians and nurses who walked with us and cared for us during the many months of treatment for Heather's cancer. Most prominent is Dr. Emily Baiyee, who consistently offered the best medicine had to offer combined with a sensitivity, gentleness, and love for Heather. Dr. Ed Ho, who first diagnosed the problem, remained a caring presence through all the time that we struggled. At the end, when all treatments were exhausted, Dr. Sunnie Kim stayed with us and made sure that all we needed we received. We could not have had a better cover of care than that offered by these stellar health care practitioners.

Numerous others read the first draft of this manuscript and provided both specific feedback to improve it and prayerful support that it would blossom into an actual book. Much thanks to Anette Punser, who knew Heather before I ever met her, Ron Arildsen, my first friend in Christ from my early days in medical school at Columbia University, and Eunice Bolden, who Heather mentored when only a teenager and now encourages me with her faith and love. John Brown read the early manuscript and offered thoughtful responses and a sensitive spirit that reminded me that my grief did not inhibit but rather enlarged my ability to communicate God's truth and love.

There are others who, before they even knew I was writing, told me that I should, which was a great reinforcement. With gratitude for Cindy Cieleski, Cheryl Fornelli, and Lenora Benda.

Harlan Van Oort was my pastor during much of this trying time. His love for Heather and I brightened my day on many occasions. I thank God for his belief in my writing and his wisdom in leading me to a publisher who would embrace me and my project. I am also grateful to my friend Jill Jones, a pastor who encouraged me regularly in prayer, especially when some of the going got tough.

I am thankful for numerous conversations with my missionary sister Peggy Giacoletto, who lost her husband a few months before I had to say goodbye to Heather, and wisely advised me to seek support through the grieving community of GriefShare.

Front Edge Publishing has been a gift from the start of the long journey that leads from writing to publication. David Crumm offered a generosity of spirit, the wisdom of experience, and highly honed gifts of editing that progressively transformed my writing into a more accessible and readable book. I was treated as a member of the family by the whole team. They embraced my work as an act of love, contributing heart, mind, and soul to the project. I am deeply grateful for all their nurture and guidance that brought hope into reality.

About the Author

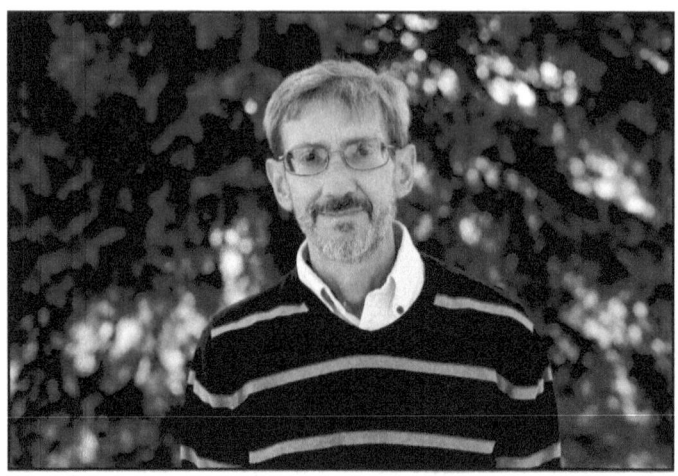

Dr. Bob Cutillo is a family physician who has worked in faith-based health care for underserved populations in the United States and abroad. He has written and taught about how a biblical view of health can reshape our culture's view of life and death, leading to a wiser and more just health care system. He is the author of *Pursuing Health in an Anxious Age*. Bob received a B.S. from Georgetown University in Washington, D.C., an M.D. from Columbia University in New York, and completed his family medicine residency at Cook County Hospital in Chicago. He has taught at several academic institutions, most recently as Associate Faculty at Denver Seminary and Assistant Clinical Professor in the Department of Family Medicine at the University of Colorado School of Medicine.

A life-long partner in mission, his cherished wife Heather died in 2023 after a three-year journey with cancer. Bob has two married children, Kate and Steve, four grandchildren, and an affectionate cat named Samwise Gamgee.

About the Author

Thank you for reading *Holding on in the Storm*. If you enjoyed reading this book, please help others discover it by leaving a review on Amazon or Goodreads. Help spread the message of *Holding on in the Storm* by sharing with friends, book clubs, and faith communities who would benefit from learning more about Dr. Bob Cutillo and his compassionate and helpful work.

Visit HoldingOnInTheStorm.com for:

- Free discussion guide download
- Additional resources
- Author information

Telling Stories In The Dark
by Jeffrey Munroe

Millions live with sorrow, trauma, and grief. Jeffrey Munroe and a national array of experts explore true stories of resiliency, hope, and faith as people transform pain and find fresh inspiration.

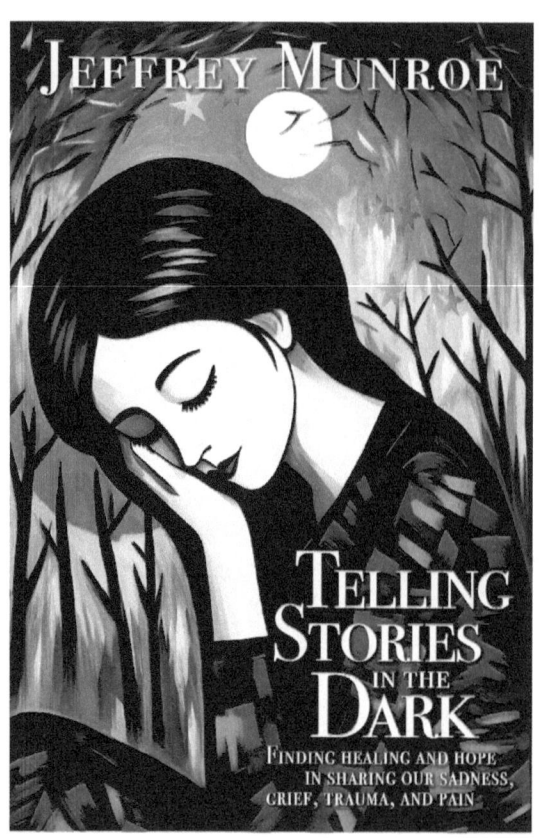

Reformed Journal Books

https://reformedjournal.com/all-books/

Never Long Enough
by Rabbi Joseph H. Krakoff

As this beautiful book moves from the darkness of grief to vibrant colors of life readers are invited to reflect on a loved one's life and legacy. An expert on grief counseling and an expert on art therapy collaborate in this unique book to be enjoyed either with a person nearing the end of life or with family and friends grieving a recent loss.

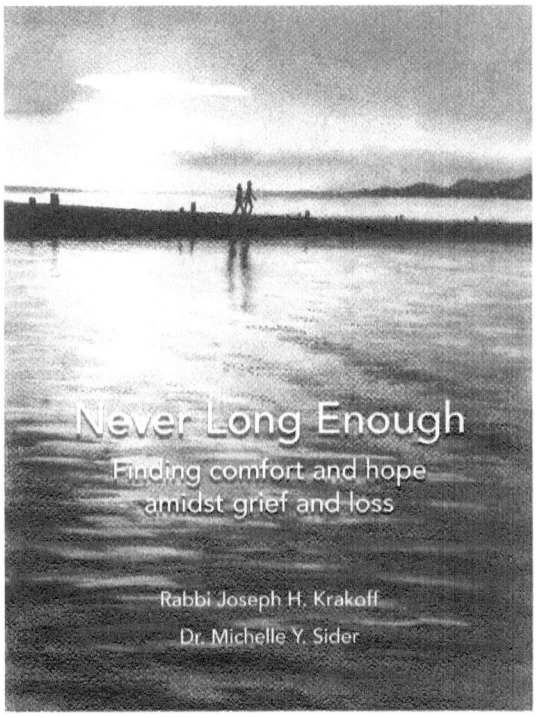

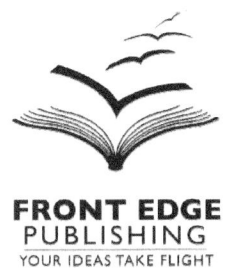

Healing a Shattered Soul
by Mindy Corporon

In *Healing a Shattered Soul*, Mindy Corporon invites readers to join her search for inspiration and hope after domestic terrorism took the lives of her father and son. Headlines about the attack circled the world. In *Healing a Shattered Soul*, Mindy takes readers inside her family's struggle, the support of their faith community and her commitment to courageous kindness.

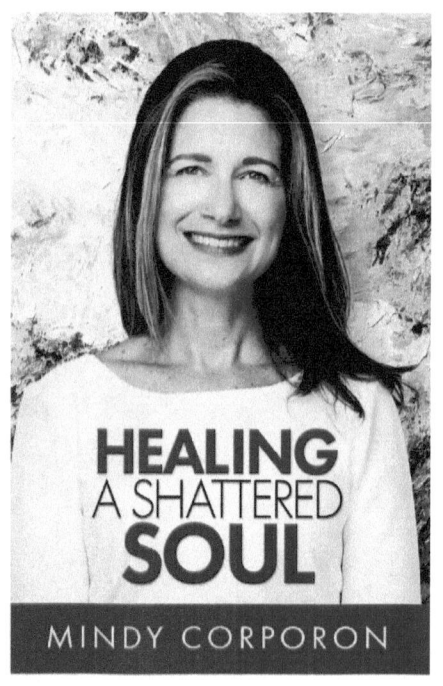

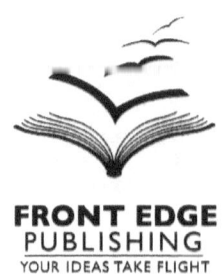

https://www.mindycorporon.com/

A Guide for Caregivers
by Benjamin Pratt

In one out of three households, someone is a caregiver: women and men who give of body, mind and soul to care for the well being of others. These millions need help, more than financial and medical assistance. They need daily, practical help in reviving their spirits and avoiding burnout. This book is drawn from the wisdom of many caregivers and we have taken their advice: these are short, easy-to-read sections packed with wisdom and practical help! Considering the millions of people worldwide who are caregivers, this book also is great for small-group study.

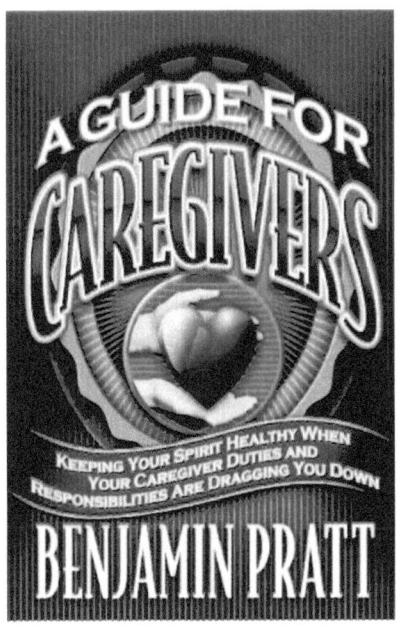

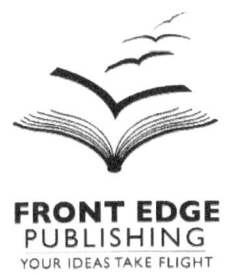

www.ingramcontent.com/pod-product-compliance
Lightning Source LLC
Chambersburg PA
CBHW020331170426
43200CB00006B/348